Prescription
Painkillers

THE LIBRARY OF ADDICTIVE DRUGS

Prescription Painkillers

HISTORY, PHARMACOLOGY, AND TREATMENT

MARVIN D. SEPPALA, M.D.
with
MARK E. ROSE, M.A.

HAZELDEN®

Hazelden
Center City, Minnesota 55012
hazelden.org

Library of Congress Cataloging-in-Publication Data
Seppala, Marvin D.
  Prescription painkillers : history, pharmacology, and treatment / Marvin D. Seppala, with Mark E. Rose.—1st ed.
      p. cm.—(The library of addictive drugs)
  Includes bibliographical references and index.
  ISBN 978-1-59285-901-6 (softcover)
  1. Analgesics. I. Rose, Mark E., 1962- II. Title. III. Series.
  RM319.S47 2010
  615'.783—dc22
                                                            2010035596

Editor's note

The names, details, and circumstances may have been changed to protect the privacy of those mentioned in this publication.

This publication is not intended as a substitute for the advice of health care professionals.

14 13 12 11 10   1 2 3 4 5 6

Cover design by Theresa Jaeger Gedig
Interior design and typesetting by Madeline Berglund

CONTENTS

INTRODUCTION

Eighty percent of the world's supply of opioid medications is used in the United States, in a country with only 4.6 percent of the world's population. This reveals the opportunity for both tremendous therapeutic advances using these medications, often simply called prescription painkillers, to address pain and suffering, as well as the potential for abuse. This quandary—that these medications are the best and basically the only available medications for moderate to severe pain and are highly reinforcing and potentially addicting—has driven clinical decision-making and government policy throughout U.S. history. The dramatic increase in prescription opioid abuse over the past fifteen years has received significant attention from diverse branches of the federal government. The Drug Enforcement Administration (DEA) has directed more resources to address issues of prescription opioid diversion; the National Institute on Drug Abuse (NIDA) has funded research to examine the appropriate treatment of prescription opioid addicts at the same time pain has become a vital sign to be used in hospitals accredited by the Joint Commission on the Accreditation of Healthcare Organizations (JCAHO) around the country; and the National Institutes of Health (NIH) has funded research into the use of these medications in the treatment of a growing medical problem—chronic pain. Despite these efforts, opioid abuse has become commonplace, and opinions vary widely on the appropriate government response, medical care, and treatment of people who are addicted to opioids.

This book provides an overview of the major aspects of the tremendous dilemma associated with the prescription opioids in the United States. Here is a chapter-by-chapter outline of the topics covered:

- Prescription opioid abuse is the fastest-growing addiction in the United States. These medications are readily available, and many people naively believe they are safe for recreational use, because they are prescribed. All of the problems and tragedies associated with opioid abuse are increasing proportionally to the increased use of the prescribed opioids. Chapter 1 documents the chilling extent of the problem.

- The historical background of opioid use and public policy in the United States is examined in chapters 2 and 3 to provide a context for understanding our current status and make sense of the federal system as it pertains to current law, oversight, and control of these medications. The medical sciences have not provided the entire framework for our policies—fear and stigma have played a major role in federal decision making regarding these medications, and continue to do so.

- In chapter 4, the availability and use of these medications will be described in a manner that links the extent of the problem to those contributing to the supply network. Some risk factors associated with the use of these medications are identical to all other drugs of abuse; others are specific to the prescribed opioids, such as treatment for pain. People obtain these medications in diverse ways. Some people see multiple physicians to obtain enough medication to maintain active addiction; others purchase medications from drug dealers who get their supplies by diversion at every step of the distribution path from the manufacturer to the physician's office. The network includes pill brokers purchasing opioids from older adults on fixed incomes, who sell some or all of their prescribed opioids, whether they need them or not, to supplement their income. Our access to these medications has changed dramatically with changing views of the treatment of pain.

- There are numerous opioids available in the United States and many routes of administration for which they are intended, resulting in many drugs available for abuse and multiple ways to use them to get high. The use of the drugs and those that are available in the United States are described in chapters 5, 6, and 7. They are most often used orally, as intended, but they can be snorted, smoked, and injected, among other means. Sometimes they must be modified for alternative use; the Internet provides quick and reliable descriptions of these methods. In chapter 8, the case of OxyContin is used to reveal how a medication thought to have a lower potential for addiction was easily altered to provide an immediate, potent high. OxyContin is also used to examine not just illicit diversion of a new opioid, but also marketing of opioid medications and controversy associated with the treatment of pain.

• Treatment for opioid addiction completes the text, in chapters 9 and 10. Opioid addiction, being the oldest drug addiction, has been treated for centuries, yet we do not have tremendous success rates (especially for heroin) and continue to have controversies. The prescribed opioids may require different treatment methods than heroin, but at this time, one can summarize by saying we have adapted treatments for heroin addiction to treat this rapidly growing problem. Perhaps that is reasonable—we're talking about opioids, not different classes of drugs—but the research is not clear about this. Prescribed opioids are commonly taken orally, but can be used intravenously, like heroin. They are smoked like heroin, and have identical effects in the brain. Some say heroin is more potent, but prescribed opioids like fentanyl and sufentanil are tremendously more powerful. The common treatment methods—maintenance and abstinence—and their attributes and shortcomings will be described. The availability of Twelve Step groups for opioid addiction is also discussed in-depth.

This book provides readers with a solid foundation regarding the multi-faceted problems associated with prescription opioids in the United States. Although the United States uses the majority of the world's prescription opioids, we are not the only country experiencing increasing problems with opioid addiction and all the regulatory questions associated with them. Knowledge of the problem provides the opportunity for healthy debate.

In my professional work, I oversee the care and treatment of people struggling with addiction, and I use that perspective to provide a broad examination of the current situation. I hope this book gives you an opportunity to learn more about this troubling, growing problem and even spurs you to become active in finding solutions.

CHAPTER 1

The Current Problem

The misuse of opioids has become a tremendous problem in the United States. Prescribed opioids are currently the fastest-growing addiction. All of the measures used to examine drug abuse reveal the incredible destruction caused by these medications. Americans have a voracious appetite for illegal drugs, and for opioid drugs in particular. As the introduction revealed, Americans make up only 4.6% of the world's population but consume 80% of the global supply of opioids; we also use 99% of the global supply of hydrocodone, and 66% of all illegal drugs (Manchikanti 2007; Califano 2007; Kuehn 2007). Retail sales of prescription opioids increased 127% between 1997 and 2006, from a total of 50.7 million grams of commonly utilized opioids (including methadone, oxycodone, fentanyl base, hydromorphone, hydrocodone, morphine, meperidine, and codeine) to 115.3 million grams. During the same time period, increases in specific prescription opioids include 196% for morphine, 244% for hydrocodone, 274% for hydromorphone, 479% for fentanyl base, 732% for oxycodone, and 1,177% for methadone (table 1.1). These figures not only underscore the massive increase in the prescribing of opioids, but also the failure of the current "war on drugs" to reduce the nation's substance abuse and addiction problem right in our own backyard (Manchikanti and Singh 2008).

Table 1.1

Retail Sales of Prescription Opioids (Grams of Medication), 1997–2006

	1997	2006	Change
Methadone	518,737	6,621,687	1,177%
Oxycodone	4,449,562	37,034,220	732%
Fentanyl Base	74,086	428,668	479%
Morphine	5,922,872	17,507,148	196%
Hydrocodone	8,669,311	29,856,368	244%
Hydromorphone	241,078	901,663	274%
Meperidine	5,765,954	4,160,033	−28%
Codeine	25,071,410	18,762,919	−25%
Total	50,713,101	115,272,706	127%

(Manchikanti and Singh 2008)

As these figures indicate, the use of prescription opioids has increased dramatically over the last decade, and nonmedical use of prescription opioids has caused increasing concern among law enforcement officials and regulatory, pain relief advocacy, and drug abuse organizations (Zacny et al. 2005). The increase in opioid abuse is particularly troubling because respiratory depression and death can result from the doses at which these drugs are frequently used, especially when mixed with other central nervous system (CNS) depressants such as alcohol and benzodiazepines (Compton and Volkow 2006). The two populations for whom prescription opioid abuse is especially troubling are adolescents, because of the uncertain implication of future addiction, and the elderly, because of increased vulnerability to toxicity. The brain is still developing until our mid-twenties, so early exposure to opioids may cause neurobiological changes and behavioral consequences that are different from what adults experience from chronic opioid use (Compton and Volkow 2006).

Figures from U.S. Government Agencies

Several U.S. government agencies have documented the pattern of increased prescription opioid use. Here are a few of the highlights from their findings:

An estimated 63 million people in the United States have used a prescription opioid for nonmedical purposes at least once during their lifetime (Woolf and Hashmi 2004). The recent peak of prescription opioid use occurred in 2004, and the numbers have leveled off since. At the peak, an estimated 4.4 million individuals age twelve or older had used prescription opioids nonmedically in the past month, according to the 2004 National Survey on Drug Use and Health (NSDUH), resulting in an estimated 158,281 emergency department visits. The opioids that were identified most frequently were oxycodone products (24.1% of opioids), hydrocodone products (23.1%), and methadone (21.3%). Among persons admitted to the emergency department for opioids, 64.6% involved the use of multiple drugs (or alcohol) (Substance Abuse and Mental Health Services Administration [SAMHSA] 2005).

Opioids now surpass marijuana as the drug class most often used by people for their first "high." In 2007, the specific drug categories with the largest number of initiates age twelve or older were prescription opioids

(2,147,000) followed by marijuana or hashish (2,090,000) (National Drug Intelligence Center [NDIC] 2009). The most recent data from NSDUH, 2008, shows that marijuana and opioids are approximately equal as the most common illicit substance for new users, but if heroin (an opioid) is added to the prescribed opioids, they easily exceed marijuana as the most common drug class to be used by people over twelve to get their first high. In 2007, 2.1% of persons age 12 or older (an estimated 5.2 million people) reported using prescription pain relievers nonmedically in the past month, a rate not significantly different from that in 2002.

The number of people who used prescription painkillers nonmedically for the first time in the past year (past-year initiates) was estimated at 2.3 million individuals (SAMHSA 2007c). The rate of past-year initiation decreased with age, with 3.8% of those age 12 to 17, 3.4% of those age 18 to 25, 0.9% of those age 26 to 34, 0.4% of those age 35 to 49, and 0.2% of those age 50 or older initiating use in the past year (SAMHSA 2007c).

The number of people seeking treatment for prescription opioid abuse has risen. The number of admissions to treatment centers for people with prescription opioids as their primary drug of choice increased 71% between 2003 and 2007, from 52,840 admissions in 2003 to 90,516 admissions in 2007. During this same period, the number of admissions to treatment centers for people with heroin as their drug of choice decreased from 273,996 in 2003 to 246,871 in 2007 (NDIC 2009).

Some prescription opioid abusers (particularly teens and young adults) switch to heroin. Prescription opioids are usually more expensive than heroin, and people abusing prescription opioids many switch to heroin because it is more affordable in many areas of the United States. OxyContin abusers with a high tolerance may use 400 milligrams of the drug daily (five 80-milligram tablets), for an average cost of $400. A comparable amount of heroin, roughly 2 grams, could be purchased at a cost of one-third to one-half that of the OxyContin (NDIC 2009).

Males age 18 and older were more likely than females to have used a prescription painkiller nonmedically in the past year (5.2% versus 4.4%). However, youths age 12 to 17, and females in all age groups were more likely than males to have used prescription opioids nonmedically in the past year (7.9% versus 6.8%). Among adults 35 and older, there were similar rates of nonmedical use of prescription pain relievers between males and females (SAMHSA 2007a). This is a dramatic shift in drug use patterns and consistent with the patterns in some states in which 12- to 17-year-old girls are drinking more frequently than their male counterparts. Historically, illicit substances are much more likely to be used by males. This change suggests a significant longer-term problem for the young women in the United States.

Definitions

Many different terms have been used by professionals, patients, and the media to describe patterns of use of prescription opioids, or painkillers. Each of these means different things to different people. Therefore, a useful place to begin our discussion of prescription painkillers is to clarify these terms.

Nonmedical use refers to using a prescription pain reliever "even once, that was not prescribed for you, or that you took only for the experience or feeling that it caused" (SAMHSA 2006c). Thus, *nonmedical use* refers to use of prescription drugs not prescribed to the user by a physician, or used only for the experience or feeling they caused (Zacny and Lichtor 2008).

Misuse refers to a patient's incorrect use of a medication, including use for other than the intended purpose, exceeding the prescribed amount, or taking the drug more frequently or for longer than prescribed (Ling, Wesson, and Smith 2005). *Misuse* and *nonmedical use* are comparable terms.

Abuse is a term that varies widely depending on the context. The Drug Enforcement Administration (DEA) defines *abuse* as the use of prescription drugs in a manner or amount inconsistent with the medical or social pattern of a culture. *Abuse* is also defined as the use of prescription medications beyond "the scope of sound medical practice" (Ling, Wesson, and Smith 2005). Abuse and misuse often overlap when referring to prescription medication. The American Psychiatric Association (APA 2000) defines *abuse* as "a maladaptive pattern of substance use, leading to clinically significant impairment or distress as manifested by one or more behaviorally based criteria." Patterns of behavior in patients who engage in the abuse of prescription opiates include escalating use, manipulation of doctors, losing prescriptions, and doctor shopping (Longo et al. 2000).

Addiction, or **substance dependence,** is the term usually used to describe the condition of someone who is hooked on a drug. *Addiction* is defined by the American Society of Addiction Medicine as a primary chronic, neurobiological disease, with genetic, psychosocial, and environmental factors influencing the development and manifestations. People with a drug addiction exhibit behaviors that include being unable to control their drug use, compulsive drug use, continued drug use despite harm, and urges and cravings for the drug (Ling, Wesson, and Smith 2005).

Physical dependence refers to neurobiological adaptation to the opioid drug from chronic exposure manifested by tolerance and withdrawal. A very important point is that physical dependence is not the same as addiction. Many patients who take a prescribed opioid for pain for an extended period will need more medication over time to relieve pain, an example of tolerance, and have opioid withdrawal symptoms if they stop abruptly, which is evidence that the body has acclimated to the constant presence of the drug. However, although many of these patients may experience some degree of drug withdrawal (also referred to as the *discontinuation syndrome),* most will not experience the overwhelming urge to recapture the drug effect and the intense drive to continue or increase the use of the drug, as is seen with addiction (Ling, Wesson, and Smith 2005).

The most widely used term to describe addiction to a prescription painkiller is **opioid dependence.** *Opioid dependence* is defined as an abnormal pattern of opiate use that leads to consequences or distress in the patient, as manifested in three or more of the following (APA 2000; Miller and Greenfield 2004):

- tolerance (the need to increase the dose to achieve the desired effect)
- withdrawal symptoms when use stops or abruptly declines
- loss of control
- persistent desire or unsuccessful attempts to cut down or control the opiate use
- preoccupation with obtaining opiate medications (such as multiple doctors, trips to the emergency department)
- important social, occupational, or recreational activities that are abandoned or reduced because of the opiate use
- continued opioid use despite awareness of adverse physical or psychological problems caused or worsened by opioids

In other words, the term *dependence* is used to describe two separate phenomena: (1) The *pharmacological* definition of drug dependence is characterized by development of tolerance and a withdrawal syndrome from prolonged use, and (2) the *psychiatric* definition of drug dependence, which is equivalent to the term drug addiction, is characterized by compulsive use, inability to reduce use, preoccupation and drug-seeking behaviors, and a heightened vulnerability to relapse after abstinence (Schwartz 1998).

Pseudo addiction describes drug-seeking behaviors in pain patients that result from inadequate pain relief, and manifest as preoccupation with and pursuit of opioid medication for pain relief, not for the drug's pleasurable effects. Pseudo-addiction develops in three phases: initially, the patient receives an inadequate level of pain relief *(analgesia),* which leads to the escalation of demands for painkillers and changes in behavior. This may be exaggerated to convince others of the pain severity and the need for more medication, which results in a crisis of mistrust between the patient and the health care team. Pseudo-addiction is preventable when the patient report of pain is accepted as valid (Ling, Wesson, and Smith 2005). The DEA recently acknowledged pseudo-addiction, in a pamphlet addressed to doctors, pharmacists, and regulators about the appropriate use of narcotics, by stating that some patients exhibiting addict-like behavior may simply be desperate for pain relief. It notes that "drug-seeking behaviors" such as visits to several doctors, requests for specific narcotics, demands for more medication, and unilateral dose escalation "cannot immediately be ascribed to addiction" and may instead be due to unrelieved pain (Sullum 2004). No single aberrant behavior can determine whether one is drug seeking secondary to pain or due to addiction. Table 1.2 provides a summary of these terms and their definitions.

Opioids are the first choice of painkiller for the relief of acute pain. They are very effective in managing moderate to severe pain, which other medications are not strong enough to handle. Opioids are also the most likely choice for treatment of *chronic pain,* defined as "pain that persists beyond the usual course of an acute disease or a reasonable time for any injury to heal that is associated with chronic pathologic processes that cause continuous pain or pain at intervals for months or years," "persistent pain that is not amenable to routine pain control methods," and "pain where healing may never occur" (Manchikanti 2006). By most definitions, chronic pain lasts at least six months. Unfortunately, medical research has not adequately proven the best treatments for chronic pain. Studies have shown significant problems with the long-term use of opioids for treatment of chronic pain (Eriksen et al. 2006).

There can be considerable overlap between the overt behavior of the person using prescription opioids and the underlying cause of that behavior. A person abusing prescription opioids daily for extended periods and a person in chronic pain taking the same opioid daily for an extended period may both become physically dependent on the opioid and experience withdrawal if they abruptly stop taking the drug. This is a physiologic

Table 1.2

Definition of Terms Related to Prescription Opioid Use, Misuse, and Dependence

Term	Definition
Addiction/substance dependence	Substance abuse involving loss of control and compulsive use of a drug despite harm
Chemical coping	Reliance on a drug for psychological stability
Diversion	Redirection of a prescription drug from its lawful purpose to illicit use; can be done with criminal intent
Misuse	Inappropriate use of a drug, whether deliberate or unintentional
Physical dependence	Condition in which ongoing use of a drug causes increased tolerance and abrupt termination causes a withdrawal syndrome
Pseudo-addiction	Condition characterized by behaviors, such as drug hoarding or demand for painkillers, that outwardly mimic addiction but is actually driven by a desire for pain relief due to undertreated pain
Self-medication	Use of a drug without consulting a health care professional to alleviate stress, depression, or anxiety
Substance abuse	Maladaptive pattern of substance use leading to considerable impairment or distress
Tolerance	Phenomenon in which pain relief or other effects of the opioid drug decrease as the body grows accustomed to a given dosage of a drug

(Passik 2009)

response to the chronic use of the medication, just as suddenly stopping a blood pressure medicine can cause hypertension, heart attack, or stroke (Lessenger and Feinberg 2008). Likewise, both an opioid abuser and a person with chronic pain that is not sufficiently treated may doctor-shop, attempt to pressure a physician into prescribing opioids (or a higher dose of an opioid), and appear to be drug seeking. Another unfortunate scenario involves a person with a history of addiction, or a person in recovery from addiction, who is experiencing significant pain and is unable to obtain appropriate medication and adequate pain relief because of a physician's fear of triggering a relapse or of being sued. If the patient's pain is under-treated, a syndrome of pseudo-addiction may occur, in which the person engages in drug-seeking behavior simply to obtain a therapeutic and effective dosage level of a pain reliever (Lessenger and Feinberg 2008). Many people in recovery from addiction describe requiring higher-than-normal levels of opioid pain medication to receive pain relief. This has not been confirmed by medical research, but altered opioid receptors could account for this form of lasting tolerance.

Mortality

In recent years, the dramatic increases in the nonmedical use of prescribed opioids have been followed by equally dramatic rises in morbidity and mortality from prescription opioids, especially in accidental overdoses and death (Streltzer, Ziegler, and Johnson 2009).

Deaths involving the use of prescription painkillers increased substantially from 2001 through 2005. The number of accidental deaths in the United States involving prescription opioids increased 114%, from approximately 3,994 in 2001 to 8,541 in 2005. Unintentional overdose deaths in which methadone was mentioned increased 220% in this time frame, from 1,158 in 2001 to 3,701 in 2005. This was primarily due to methadone used for the treatment of pain, not for maintenance treatment of heroin addiction. Also, the number of accidental deaths from prescription opioids surpassed the number of accidental deaths from cocaine and heroin throughout this period (NDIC 2009).

Six states (Maine, New Hampshire, Vermont, Maryland, Utah, and New Mexico) participate in the mortality component of the Drug Abuse Warning Network (DAWN). Among these states, the death rates from opioid-related drug misuse in 2003 ranged from 7.2 per 100,000 population in New Hampshire to 11.6 per 100,000 population in New Mexico. In all six of these states, most deaths related to opioid abuse involved multiple drugs. In five of the six states, adults age 35 to 54 had the highest rates of opioid misuse deaths. In the remaining state (Maine), the highest rate was for adults age 21 to 34 (SAMHSA 2006b).

Fatalities associated with prescription opioid use are strongly linked to the simultaneous use of multiple substances. An examination of 2,024 opiate-related deaths in England examined the factors associated with the deaths of both non-addicts and addicts in the group. The non-addicts tended to be older than 45 and died as a result of intentional overdose, while the addicts tended to be young males and victims of accidental overdose. In 93% of the deaths, opioids were used in combination with another substance. Among the non-addicts, alcohol was used most often in accidental deaths and antidepressants were typically used in the intentional deaths. Likewise, illicit drugs and hypnotics/sedatives were typically reported in the accidental deaths among the addicts (Schifano et al. 2006).

A national epidemic of drug-related deaths in the United States began in the 1990s, coinciding with the increased prescribing of opioid painkillers. National figures from the Centers for Disease Control and prescription painkiller sales data from the DEA found that unintentional drug overdose mortality rates increased an average of 5.3% per year from 1979 to 1990, and 18.1% per year from 1990 to 2002. The rapid increase during the 1990s reflects the rising number of deaths attributed to opioids and unspecified drugs. Between 1999 and 2002, the number of prescription opioid overdoses, or poisonings, that were indicated on death certificates increased by 91.2%, while heroin and cocaine poisonings increased 12.4% and 22.8%, respectively. By 2002, prescription opioid poisoning was listed in 5,528 deaths—more than either heroin or cocaine. The increase in deaths generally matched the increase in sales for each type of prescription opioid, and the increase in deaths involving methadone paralleled the increase in methadone used as a painkiller rather than methadone used in narcotic treatment programs (Paulozzi, Budnitz, and Xi 2006).

Some regions of the United States have been especially hard hit by the increase in prescription opioid-related overdose deaths. In rural Virginia, drug overdose deaths increased 300% from 1997 to 2003, with 58% of these deaths due to the use of multiple drugs. Prescription opioids (74.0%), antidepressants (49.0%), and benzodiazepines (39.3%) were found more often among the deceased than illicit drugs. Two-thirds of the deceased were 35 to 54 years old and 37% were female (Wunsch et al. 2009).

Methadone-related Mortality

Methadone is a safe and effective drug when it is properly used for pain or as treatment for opioid addiction, but it can be deadly when it is prescribed by those unfamiliar with its use, or is misused or abused, particularly when taken with other prescription drugs, street drugs, or alcohol. Although much concern has been raised over methadone clinics being the primary source of abused methadone, most methadone-related deaths involve the abuse or misuse of methadone originating from hospitals, pharmacies, practitioners, and pain management physicians. From 1999 to 2005, the number of methadone-related deaths increased more than fivefold, from 786 to 4,462, a rate higher than overdose deaths associated with other prescription opioids such as oxycodone, hydrocodone, and fentanyl (U.S. General Accounting Office [USGAO] 2009). By comparison, deaths associated with other prescription opioids such as oxycodone, morphine, hydromorphone, and hydrocodone increased 90% from 1999 to 2004 (table 1.3) (NDIC 2007).

In 2004, the Substance Abuse and Mental Health Services Administration (SAMHSA) performed a national assessment to help understand the causes of this increase in methadone-related deaths. The report concluded that most deaths involved one of three scenarios:

- the accumulation of toxic levels of methadone during the initiation phase of methadone maintenance treatment, or from methadone prescribed for pain management that was due to a combination of overestimating the ability of the patient to tolerate methadone and methadone's long and variable half-life
- the misuse of diverted methadone by individuals with little or

Table 1.3

Deaths Associated with Methadone versus Other Opioids, 1999–2004

Year	Methadone	Other prescription opioids
1999	786	2,757
2000	988	2,932
2001	1,456	3,484
2002	2,360	4,431
2003	2,974	4,877
2004	3,849	5,242
Change from 1999 to 2004	390%	90%

(NDIC 2007)

no opioid tolerance who may have taken excessive doses in an attempt to achieve euphoria

• the additive or synergistic effects of methadone in combination with other central nervous system depressants (alcohol, benzodi-azepines, or other prescription opioids) among individuals with little or no tolerance to opiates

Medwatch, the Food and Drug Administration's safety information and adverse event reporting program, reported that seizures of methadone tablets (prescribed to treat pain) increased 133% between 2001 and 2002, in contrast to seizures of liquid methadone (dispensed to treat opioid addiction), which increased 11% during the same period (Center for

Substance Abuse Treatment [CSAT] 2004b). From 1994 to 2001, DAWN reported substantial increases in drug-related emergency department visits for several prescription painkillers, including 352% for oxycodone, 230% for methadone, and 131% for hydrocodone (SAMHSA 2004; Manchikanti 2006).

Methadone is more likely to cause overdose because of the slow rate at which it is broken down in the body. This can contribute to increased blood levels, increased toxicity, and respiratory depression, which can cause death. Methadone prescriptions for pain management grew from about 531,000 in 1998 to about 4.1 million in 2006, an increase of almost 700% (USGAO 2009), and since the late 1990s, methadone has been increasingly prescribed by practitioners to treat pain. It is a relatively inexpensive, long-lasting pain medication, therefore very useful. Using methadone to treat pain is very different from using it to treat opioid addiction. While a single dose of methadone suppresses opioid withdrawal symptoms for a day or more, it generally relieves pain for only four to eight hours despite remaining in the body much longer. It may also take three to five days to achieve full pain relief, so dosage increases must be done more slowly than with other opioids. As a result, patients may take too much methadone before the previous dose has left the body. However, if taken too often, in too high a dose, or with certain other medicines or supplements, it may build up in the body to a toxic level. Variability in methadone's absorption, metabolism, and relative pain-relief potency among patients requires a highly individualized approach to prescribing by an experienced physician (USGAO 2009).

From 2002 to 2007, the distribution of methadone to businesses associated with pain management such as pharmacies and practitioners almost tripled, increasing from about 2.3 millions grams to about 6.5 million grams. In contrast, distribution to methadone clinics increased more slowly, from about 5.3 million grams to about 6.5 million grams (USGAO 2009). Although the distribution of methadone for pain management is largely responsible for the increases in methadone-related deaths, methadone clinics do contribute to a fair amount of diversion and a significant proportion of the deaths. Perhaps the biggest reason underlying these increases in deaths among methadone clinic patients has to do with methadone clinics offering methadone maintenance therapy to anyone who meets a loose criteria of opioid dependence. In this respect, many of the patients are very different from the traditional methadone clinic patient who has a history of chronic heroin addiction and a correspondingly high tolerance to opioid drugs. Methadone clinics usually escalate the dose of methadone during the induction phase of therapy, and the majority of the rare methadone clinic-associated fatalities occur during this induction phase of treatment. Methadone clinic personnel may overestimate the degree of opioid tolerance in the patient, or a patient may use other opioids or CNS depressant drugs in addition to the prescribed methadone (CSAT 2004b; Manchikanti 2006). Table 1.4 summarizes the increases in the legitimate distribution of methadone from 2001 to 2006.

Table 1.4

Legitimate Methadone Distribution, in Grams, 2001–2006

Year	Practitioners	Pharmacists	Hospitals
2001	6,250	1,660,432	225,368
2002	10,381	2,328,287	310,027
2003	15,113	3,274,059	393,957
2004	35,466	4,228,660	466,028
2005	43,199	4,810,467	509,138
2006	51,046	5,986,488	584,144
Change from 2001 to 2006	715%	261%	159%

(NDIC 2007)

CHAPTER 2

The History of Opioids

The current epidemic in nonmedical use of prescription opioids is actually part of a recurring pattern, and we can learn valuable lessons by studying the history of these drugs. The extensive consumption of opioids, including morphine and heroin, as well as the massive consumption of cocaine, which occurred before World War I, are now all but forgotten. We assume that recent epidemics—heroin in the 1960s and 1970s, cocaine in the 1980s, or prescription painkillers today—are new phenomena. The history of attempts at legislative control in the United States, and their successes and failures, suggests that devising and implementing a rational approach for the current problem is more likely to occur if we consider these earlier efforts at narcotic regulation (Musto 1999).

Opioid Use throughout History

Opium is derived from the juices of the poppy plant *Papaver somniferum*. The word *opium* comes from *opos*, the Greek word for *juice*. Opioid is used as an umbrella term for all the natural and synthetic (humanmade) medicines that are derived from or based on opium. Opiate, a more commonly used term, applies only to those medicines that specifically use opium or thebaine, the natural products of the opium poppy—they are the "natural" opioids. The natural medications and the synthetics act the same way in the brain.

The medicinal and recreational use of opium dates back to antiquity. Evidence of poppy plant use from preserved remains of cultivated poppy seeds and pods dates back to the fourth millennium BCE (Booth 1996). The Sumerians (4000 BCE) and the Egyptians (2000 BCE) knew of the pain-relieving and euphoric effects of the poppy plant (Rehman 2001). Opium was proposed as a remedy for numerous ailments in the Ebers papyrus, an ancient Egyptian medical document, dating from about 1550 BCE. The recreational use of opium in ancient central Asia was mentioned by the Greek historian Herodotus in the fifth century BCE, when he observed that the Massagets (a people who inhabited the northern coast of the Caspian Sea) inhaled the smoke from burnt poppy heads to induce euphoria (Ulyankina 1987; Smith 2008).

In 1732, British physician Thomas Dover developed "Dover's Powder," a formula that combined opium with ipecacuanha (known today as ipecac), which induces vomiting. The result was a pain-reducing potion that could cause euphoria but could not be ingested in large quantities because of its emetic properties. It was taken as a nonprescription medicine for more than 200 years and was also prescribed by physicians until the early 1900s when its addictive properties were realized (Boyes 1931).

The publication of Thomas de Quincey's *Confessions of an English Opium-Eater* (1821–1822) brought the addictive potential of opioids (which was already known) into the spotlight (Smith 2008).

Enter Morphine

Drugs have been used for millennia in their natural form. Coca leaves and poppy plants were chewed, dissolved in alcoholic beverages, or taken in some way that diluted the impact of the active agent (Musto 1991). Advances in chemistry in the nineteenth century spawned the modern pharmaceutical industry, and this industry quickly turned its attention to the old botanical products already in wide use. These agents were reprocessed and made more widely available in highly refined and far more potent forms—among them morphine and heroin (refined from opium poppies) and cocaine (from coca leaves) (Drucker 2000).

Morphine was discovered in 1803 by Friedrich Wilhelm Adam Sertürner (1783–1841), an obscure, uneducated, 20-year-old pharmacist's assistant with little experience but lots of curiosity. Sertürner was curious about the medicinal properties of opium and managed to isolate an organic alkaloid compound from the resinous gum secreted by the opium poppy. What followed was the first recorded use of morphine in history; Sertürner and three of his friends each ingested a staggering amount of 90 mg of the morphine (in three divided doses) over forty-five minutes. Sertürner had to induce vomiting to try to control the ensuing abdominal pains and sleepiness. Following this initial rocky experience with morphine, he performed a series of experiments in his spare time, often on himself, to learn about its therapeutic effects and potential hazards. The results were published in a letter to a pharmacy journal in 1805, but his work was initially ignored (Bause 2009). Sertürner persevered with his groundbreaking research and found that opium with the alkaloid removed had no effect on animals, but the alkaloid itself had ten times the power of processed opium. He named the substance morphine, after Morpheus, the Greek god of dreams, because of its tendency to induce sleep (Schmitz 1985; Musto 1999). In 1817, he presented the scientific community, and the rest of the world, with the "crystallizable" isolate of opium in the journal *Annalen der Physik*. Sertürner's crystallization of morphine was the first isolation of a natural plant alkaloid, and had the effect of launching the study of alkaloid chemistry and the emergence of the modern pharmaceutical industry (Bause 2009; Musto 1999).

In 1818, French physician François Magendie published a paper that described how morphine brought pain relief and much-needed sleep to an ailing young girl. This paper stimulated widespread medical interest, and by the mid-1820s morphine was widely available in western Europe from several sources, including the Darmstadt chemical company started by Heinrich Emanuel Merck.

From its earliest application, morphine has been used for pain relief and is still considered the standard by which all other pain-relieving drugs are measured. Physicians believed the new opium derivative to be non-addicting, and hoped that it could actually cure opium addiction in patients. Doctors prescribed the new opiate often.

Opium Comes to America

Opium was brought to North America by European explorers and settlers. The colonists regarded opium as a valuable resource for pain relief. Benjamin Franklin regularly took laudanum (opium extract in alcohol) to alleviate kidney stone pain during the final years of his life. Opium poppies were grown legally. In a letter to a Pennsylvania farmer on August 24, 1781, Philadelphia physician Thomas Bond wrote: "The opium you sent is pure and of good quality. I hope you will take care of the seed" (O'Donnell 1969). During the War of 1812, opium was scarce, but "some parties produced it in New Hampshire and sold the product at $10 to $12 per pound" (O'Donnell 1969).

Americans also recognized the potential hazard from continuous opium use long before the availability of morphine and hypodermic syringes. The American Dispensatory of 1818 noted that habitual use of opium could lead to "tremors, paralysis, stupidity and general emaciation." However, this cautionary note was balanced by proclamations of the extraordinary value of opium for a multitude of ailments ranging from cholera to asthma. Considering that medical treatments of the day included blistering, vomiting, and bleeding, it's not hard to understand why opium was as cherished by patients as it was by their physicians (Musto 1991).

Opiate Use in Nineteenth-century America

The United States during the nineteenth century can best be described as a "dope fiend's paradise" (Brecher 1972). Opium was legally imported and sold throughout the century, and morphine was legally manufactured domestically from the imported opium (O'Donnell 1969). Opium was sold in a crude form containing about 10% morphine, as well as in concoctions derived from crude opium such as paregoric, laudanum, and a solution in acetic acid known as "black drop."

Physicians in the nineteenth century prescribed opiates for pain, as they do now, and for cough, diarrhea, dysentery, and a host of other illnesses. Physicians often referred to opium and morphine as "G.O.M."—"God's own medicine." Dr. H. H. Kane's 1880 textbook listed fifty-four diseases that benefited from morphine injections, including anemia, angina pectoris, diabetes, insanity, nymphomania, ovarian neuralgia, tetanus, vaginismus, and vomiting associated with pregnancy (Kane 1880).

Dr. J. R. Black's 1889 view that an opiate "calms in place of exciting the baser passions" was very widely agreed upon and was the basis for the widespread use of opiates as tranquilizers. Dr. Horatio Day described the tranquilizing role of the opiates in *The Opium Habit* (1868), three years after the close of the Civil War: "Maimed and shattered survivors from a hundred battlefields, diseased and disabled soldiers released from hostile prisons, anguished and hopeless wives and mothers, made so by the slaughter of those who were dearest to them, have found, many of them, temporary relief from their sufferings in opium" (Day 1868). Compare this to the increasing use of opioids to treat our veterans returning from the Middle East.

Indeed, morphine was a frequently used painkiller during the Civil War. After the war, addiction to morphine among veterans was so great that morphine addiction became known as "soldier's disease" (Casey 1978).

Another nineteenth-century use of opiates was as a substitute for alcohol. As Dr. J. R. Black explained in a paper titled "Advantages of Substituting the Morphia Habit for the Incurably Alcoholic," published in the *Cincinnati Lancet-Clinic* in 1889, morphine "is less inimical to healthy life than alcohol." It "is less productive of acts of violence and crime; in short . . . the use of morphine in place of alcohol is but a choice of evils, and by far the lesser" (Black 1889). Then he continued: "On the score of economy the morphine habit is by far the better. The regular whiskey drinker can be made content in his craving for stimulation, at least for quite a long time, on two or three grains of morphine a day, divided into appropriate portions, and given at regular intervals. If purchased by the drachm at fifty cents this will last him twenty days. Now it is safe to say that a like amount of spirits for the steady drinker cannot be purchased for two and one half cents a day, and that the majority of them spend five and ten times that sum a day as a regular thing." Many physicians did in fact convert alcoholics to morphine, and in Kentucky, this practice did not die out among older physicians until the late 1930s or early 1940s (Brecher 1972).

The nineteenth-century distribution of opiates extended beyond the large cities into towns, villages, and hamlets. A New England physician-druggist wrote around 1870: "In this town I began business twenty years since. The population then at 10,000 has increased only inconsiderably, but my sales have advanced from 50 pounds of opium the first year to 300 pounds now; and of laudanum [opium in alcohol] four times upon what was formerly required. About 50 regular purchasers come to my shop, and as many more, perhaps, are divided among the other three apothecaries in the place. Some country dealers also have their quota of dependents" (Brotman and Freedman 1968).

Another significant development by mid-century was perfection of the hypodermic syringe. By 1870, it had become a familiar instrument to American physicians and patients (Howard-Jones 1971). Prevalent medical opinion held that the addiction process occurred in the individual's stomach and that ingestion of an opiate was responsible for addiction. The hypodermic needle and syringe were greeted as a boon by physicians who hoped to use morphine injections to kill pain, believing that the injection process itself would eliminate the addiction problem (Levine 1974; Casey 1978). The reusable hypodermic needle was first used in 1855. It is primarily attributed to Dr. Alexander Wood of Edinburgh, Scotland. Initially it was used to inject subcutaneously, but this changed quickly to intravenous. Other than opioids, very few medications were available for such use. With this new route of administration a quantum leap in intoxication could be attained. Unfortunately, Wood and his wife became addicted to morphine. By the Civil War, morphine injection was common and helpful in the relief of severe pain (Karch 1998).

Patent Medicines

Throughout the late 1800s, opiates and countless pharmaceutical preparations containing them "were as freely accessible as aspirin is today" (Schmitz 1985), and were available through five legal channels: by prescription, over the counter at drugstores, at grocery and general stores, through mail order, and from innumerable patent medicines (Brecher 1972).

The term *patent medicine* described all prepackaged medicines sold over-the-counter without a doctor's prescription, and the second half of the nineteenth century is considered the golden age of American patent medicines. Rapid increases in industry and manufacturing, urban living, advertising in national newspapers and magazines, and the absence of drug regulation all contributed to a boom in the production and consumption of patent medicines. Many people turned to patent medicines out of fear and distrust of contemporary medical practices, which is understandable considering the methods in common practice during that era such as bloodletting, the use of harsh purgatives, and emetics. Before the advent of germ theory at the end of the nineteenth century, physicians had very few therapies that could compete with the patent medicine industry's promise of symptom relief or cure in a bottle (Smithsonian National Museum of American History).

Americans could obtain opium and morphine whenever they wanted, for whatever reason they chose, from an over-the-counter or mail-order catalog purchase. Patent medicine companies were the leading advertisers in American newspapers. They developed a clever protection from prying investigations or public pressure to reveal secret formulas, or from any state requirement to make only valid claims for effectiveness: The proprietary manufacturers included in their lucrative contracts with newspapers a condition that the advertising agreement would be void if the state in which the newspaper was published passed any laws affecting the sale or manufacture of the nostrums (Berridge and Edwards 1981; Musto 1999).

In the nation's capital, the manufacturers also fought off requirements that their nostrums be correctly labeled as to the contents. Bills to enact such a law under the interstate commerce clause of the Constitution were defeated repeatedly, but in the 1890s a new reforming spirit was evident in the nation. The simplest reform, correct labeling, was part of the Pure Food and Drug Act of 1906, which stipulated that any over-the-counter or "patent" medicine disclose the inclusion of morphine, cocaine, cannabis, or chloral hydrate. Widely read magazines such as *Collier's* and *Ladies Home Journal* railed against patent medicines, especially against morphine and cocaine, even after passage of the truth-in-labeling laws, and the exposés and negative press continued unabated until the next major step, which was restriction on the availability of the drugs themselves (Musto 1999).

Patent medicines were aggressively marketed, and before the beginning of federal drug regulation in 1906, patent medicine manufacturers made any therapeutic claims for their products that they wished. In 1905 and 1906, *Collier's* magazine ran a series of influential articles exposing the deceptive and unsafe methods practiced by these manufacturers. Such exposés promoted the first federal Food and Drug Act, signed into law by President Theodore Roosevelt on June 30, 1906, which required drug labeling to include a list of ingredients and prohibited manufacturers from making false and misleading claims (Smithsonian National Museum of American History).

By the end of the nineteenth century, millions of Americans were regularly using patent medicines, tonics, salves, potions, and commercially available beverages containing combinations of opium, morphine, cocaine, and alcohol (Berridge and Edwards 1987; Courtwright 1985; Musto 1987). These substances were the frontline medicines of the time and almost universally prescribed by doctors and sold over the counter. Their psychoactive properties were also well recognized and exploited to relieve sleep disturbances, anxiety, and depression. These drugs were among the few effective tools of early medical practice, were aggressively marketed, and quickly developed huge markets because few alternative therapies were available and because they had a powerful effect on symptoms. However, with increasingly widespread use of these powerful drugs came the growing awareness of their addictive potential (Drucker 2000).

Throughout the late 1800s, physicians commonly prescribed opium and morphine for menstrual and menopausal disorders, and opiate patent medicines were extravagantly advertised as having the ability to relieve "female troubles" (Casey 1978). Women had become the prevalent class of opiate users, and the prescribing of patent medicines containing opiates to women was accepted without question. The sentiment was that the opiates were a convenient, genteel drug for a dependent lady who would never be seen drinking in public; this tacit acceptance of opiate use by women and simultaneous stigmatization of drinking by women contributed to the excess of women among opiate users (Brecher 1972).

In addition to a preponderance of opiate users being female during the last part of the nineteenth century, there is evidence that users were older in age. An 1880 Chicago survey of opiate users found an average age for males of 41.4 years and 39.4 years for females. An 1885 Iowa survey similarly noted that the majority of opiate users were found among the educated and higher socioeconomic levels of society (Brecher 1972).

The Introduction of Heroin

In the late nineteenth century, it was believed that if the "addictive" properties of opium could be filtered out, its therapeutic essence could be captured. Diacetylmorphine was first synthesized from morphine in 1874 by simply adding two acetyl groups. This drug is roughly three times more potent than morphine, with a more rapid onset of action. Heinrich Dreser, in charge of drug development at the Bayer Company in Germany, tested the new semisynthetic drug on animals, on humans, and most notably, on himself. Dreser was impressed. Contrary to common opinion, heroin was not created to treat morphine or opium addiction, but rather was developed and marketed to fill the desperate need for a powerful cough suppressant. The leading causes of death at that time—tuberculosis and pneumonia—were linked to uncontrollable coughing, and the drug per-formed well in preliminary testing by the manufacturer. Dreser declared diacetylmorphine to be an effective treatment for a variety of respiratory ailments, especially bronchitis, asthma, and tuberculosis.

In 1898, the Bayer Company introduced diacetylmorphine, under the brand name of Heroin, to the commercial market in Europe and the United States. The new wonder drug enjoyed widespread acceptance in the medical profession, and Bayer was enthusiastically selling Heroin in dozens of countries. Free samples were handed out to physicians, and the medical profession remained largely unaware of the addiction potential for years. Ultimately, Bayer halted production of Heroin in 1913; by that time, the notoriety surrounding the drug was such that the company eliminated any mention of Heroin from the official company history (Musto 1974; Musto 1999).

The use of heroin in the United States prior to 1916 was essentially unrestricted, and by 1912 in New York City it had replaced morphine as the drug of choice among young males, according to Bellevue Hospital records. The addictive nature of heroin had been recognized rather quickly, with the American Medical Association (AMA) issuing a warning in 1902.

Heroin was popular because it could be inhaled by sniffing, like cocaine, as well as injected by hypodermic syringes. When injected into the bloodstream, heroin crossed the blood-brain barrier more quickly than morphine and therefore gave a more intense high. During the years of intense concern over social control, which began with the First World War, heroin became linked with gang violence and criminal activity. Some believed that heroin stimulated the user to commit crimes or at least provided the courage to engage in bank robberies or muggings. By the early 1920s most of the crime in New York City was blamed on drug use, chiefly the opiates, including heroin (Kuhne 1926; Musto 1999).

The preference for heroin over morphine among recreational users, and the belief that other opiates could fulfill heroin's role as a painkiller and cough suppressant, led to a move to ban heroin for medical purposes. The heroin problem also contributed to an American fear of foreign nations after World War I, because the drug was manufactured in other countries and smuggled into the United States. The Swiss drug industry, for example, produced large amounts of heroin that found its way into the United States. Heroin's image as a foreign product that was popular with feared domestic groups helped support an isolationist stance (Musto 1999).

The Extent and Growing Problem of Opiate Use

During the nineteenth century, narcotics were largely unregulated in the United States, were freely available, and were widely used. Although some states had laws governing the sale of narcotics, and many municipalities forbade opium smoking to suppress the practice among recent immigrants from China, these laws were only sporadically enforced. In practice just about anyone could easily obtain pure drugs at a modest cost. Pharmacists even delivered drugs, dispatching messenger boys with vials of morphine for home delivery. Some customers were actually unaware they were ingesting opiates and cocaine because patent medicine proprietors slipped narcotics into their products without describing the ingredients, a practice which became illegal in 1906 when truth-in-labeling laws were first passed. Additionally, doctors frequently overprescribed narcotics. Opiates were among the few effective drugs they possessed, and the temptation was overwhelming to alleviate the symptoms (and thus continue the patronage) of their patients, especially those who were seriously or chronically ill (Courtwright 2001).

The extent that opiates were prescribed is illustrated in an 1886 survey of 10,000 prescriptions filled by thirty-five Boston drugstores—1,481 of them contained opiates. Among prescriptions refilled three or more times, 78% contained opiates (Pepper 1886). An 1883–1885 survey of the state of Iowa, which then had a population of less than 2 million, found 3,000 stores where opiates were sold (Terry and Pellens 1928). Also, one wholesale drug house was believed to distribute more than 600 proprietary medicines and other products containing opiates (Towns 1912).

During the nineteenth century, the annual per capita consumption of opiates rose steadily from about 12 grains in 1840 (an average single dose is 1 grain) to 52 grains by the mid-1890s. Then the average individual consumption gradually subsided up to 1914, by which time the per capita rate had fallen back to the level of about 1880 (Musto 1999).

Widespread opiate addiction was first documented in the United States following the Civil War, occurring, as mentioned earlier, as the result of opiates administered to large numbers of injured soldiers. Opiate addiction in the United States peaked about the turn of the century, when the number of people addicted to the drug was close to 300,000 out of a population of 76 million, plus an unknown number of irregular users, a rate of opiate addiction that has never since been equaled or surpassed in the United States (Musto 1999; Courtwright 1982).

Opiate addiction was not entirely ignored by the medical profession. As the number of addicts increased in the 1870s and 1880s, some physicians began to specialize in treating addiction and developing theories of addiction. There was debate over the cause of addiction: whether it, along with alcoholism, was symptomatic of a more general neurological disorder; whether gradual or rapid withdrawal was preferable; whether withdrawal could or should be alleviated with non-narcotic drugs and, if so, which ones. A hundred years later, most of these issues are still not completely resolved (Courtwright 2001).

SUMMARY

Opiates were the first, and for centuries the only, effective medications known to human beings. They continue to be the most effective pain medications available. History reveals their addictive potential, and when opioids are readily available, addiction rates increase. Much can be learned from the excessive rates of opioid addiction in the late 1800s, when opioids were readily available by prescription and via patent medicines. We are in the midst of another opioid epidemic, secondary to increased access to these powerful medications, causing remarkably similar though more devastating problems. Ultimately the opioid epidemic of the 1800s was addressed by the federal government.

Early Regulation and Treatment

Nineteenth-century physicians interested in addiction were limited by the embryonic state of medical science, and although many key discoveries had not yet been made, such as the existence of brain receptors, endorphins, or opioid antagonists, the absence of any regulatory body allowed considerable latitude for experimentation with ways to treat opiate addiction. Some medical specialists believed that addiction and alcoholism were the interrelated manifestations of a common underlying nervous disorder termed *inebriety,* and that "inebriates" needed institutional care (Courtwright 2001).

Changing Attitudes toward Opiate Use and Addiction

The nonmedicinal use of opiates, while legal in both the United States and England, was not considered respectable during the nineteenth century. As a perceptive American writer noted in the *Catholic World* in 1881 (Anonymous 1881), opiates were as disreputable as drinking alcoholic beverages—and much harder to detect (Brecher 1972). Opiate use was also frowned upon in some social circles as an immoral vice comparable to dancing, smoking, theater-going, gambling, or sexual promiscuity. But while deemed immoral, opiate use in the nineteenth century was not subject to the same moral sanctions currently practiced.

Our nineteenth-century forebears correctly saw that the major problem of opiates was their potential for abuse and dependence. Although the word *addiction* was seldom used in the nineteenth century, the phenomenon was well understood, with the true nature of the narcotic evil becoming visible, as an article in the *Catholic World* pointed out, when someone who has been using an opiate for some time attempts to quit (Anonymous 1881). At the time, people also perceived opiate use as a "will-weakening" vice, believing opiate users with a strong will could stop if they tried hard enough. It was well known that addicts deprived of their opiates would lie or steal to get their drug, and that addicts "cured" of their addiction repeatedly relapsed. Thus, there was much discussion about the moral degeneration caused by the opiates. However, there was very little support for a law banning these substances. The reason for this lack of demand for opiate prohibition was very simple: the drugs were not viewed as a menace to society (Brecher 1972).

As mentioned, opium was available in many forms derived from crude opium long before the nineteenth century. In the United States, the two developments that spurred both widespread use and concern about opiates were the isolation of morphine and its injection into the body with hypodermic syringes, and the introduction of smoking opium by a feared minority, the Chinese (Musto 1999). The more intense high produced by intravenous use of morphine and opium introduced U.S. culture to a more dangerous form of opioid addiction. The recognition and fear associated with evidence of a worse form of opioid addiction—much like the more recent experience with crack cocaine compared to snorted cocaine—contributed significantly to the cultural shift in perception of the opioid addict and to how the U.S. government responded. Stigma, fear, and lack of accurate information about drug addiction as a disease have contributed to the U.S. response to addictive drugs.

The later part of the nineteenth century also marked the beginning of a popular revulsion at the problem of addiction and a growing demonization of drugs and the people who became addicted to them. These sentiments were fueled, in part, by the lurid pulp journalism of the late

Victorian age, with its overheated moralistic tales of "enslavement and depravity" associated with drug use, often with racial stereotypes of drug users (such as the Chinese and opium). It was also a period of moral crusading aimed at eradicating all varieties of "sinful" behavior from American society, complicated by the fact that these moral campaigns were part of a powerful and mostly positive historical movement of the Progressive era that promoted social betterment and public health (Courtwright 2001).

Within twenty-five years, attitudes toward addiction had dramatically changed. Even as the country was having second thoughts about alcohol prohibition, there was virtual consensus on the need to suppress narcotic addiction. Some extremists in the 1920s and 1930s even proposed firing squads as a permanent solution for the drug addiction problem, on the theory that the only cured addict was a dead one. This pronounced attitudinal shift was partially related to the changing perceptions of who drug addicts were, how they acquired their habits, and how they behaved under the influence of drugs. Addiction thus went from being regarded as the pathetic condition of a sick person in need of proper treatment to a stigmatized condition among social outcasts and members of undesirable groups who needed punishment (Courtwright 2001).

The Government Gets Involved

U.S. narcotic policy has been highly variable, having passed through at least four major stages during the past 100 years. In the nineteenth and early twentieth centuries, government involvement was minimal. Drug use was largely a private matter, as was drug treatment. Addiction was understood as either a personal or a medical problem, and various treatments were provided on a fee-for-service basis. From 1909 to 1923 the federal government became increasingly involved in the matter of addiction, as a series of important laws, court cases, and administrative decisions effectively criminalized nonmedical narcotic use and dictated specific treatments such as long-term maintenance and detoxification. The following four decades, from 1923 to 1965, have been described as the classic era of narcotic control in the sense of the simple, consistent, and rigid approach by the government. Few resources for treatment were available to addicts, and U.S. narcotic policy was strict and punitive, both in comparison with other Western countries and with the preceding era in American history. During the 1960s the harshly punitive approach was challenged and gradually superseded by a hybrid approach that combined traditional law enforcement with new treatment strategies such as methadone maintenance and therapeutic communities (Courtwright 2001).

The First Laws

In 1872, California passed the first anti-opium law, which stated that "the administration of laudanum, an opium preparation, or any other narcotic to any person with the intent thereby to facilitate the commission of a felony" now constituted a felony (Levine 1974). However, this first awkward attempt failed to control opium use. In 1881, the California legislature passed a law making it a misdemeanor to maintain a place where opium was sold, given away, or smoked. The bill applied only to commercial locations, and specifically to opium dens. Smoking opium alone, or with friends in a private residence, was not covered by the legislation, and the practice continued. In the same year, California became the first state to establish a separate bureau of narcotic enforcement, and was one of the first states to treat addicts. In 1874, Connecticut became the first state to pass a law declaring the "narcotic addict" incompetent to attend to his or her personal affairs. Commitment to a state insane asylum for "medical care and treatment" was mandated until the patient was "cured" of the "addiction" (Levine 1974).

In general, legislative attempts to control narcotic drugs during the nineteenth century were thwarted because the federal government had no practical control over the health professions, there were no representative national health organizations to aid the government in drafting regulations, and there was a total absence of controls on the labeling, composition, and advertising of compounds that might contain opiates or cocaine. States were responsible for medicine and medical care, limiting federal intervention. The free-market economy of the United States meant complete lack of restraint at every level, from preparation to consumption of opiate drugs (Musto 1999).

The Pure Food and Drug Act of 1906

Overcoming years of resistance by patent medicine manufacturers, the federal government enacted the Pure Food and Drug Act in 1906. This act did not prevent sales of addictive drugs like opiates and cocaine, but it did require accurate labeling for all patent remedies sold in interstate commerce. After the act was passed, the manufacturers of Coca-Cola— which was introduced in 1886 as a drink offering the advantages of cocaine but without the danger of alcohol (Musto 1991)—stopped using unprocessed coca leaves containing cocaine, substituting decocainized leaves to keep the same flavor; caffeine remained in the beverage as a stimulant (Casey 1978). Subsequent amendments to the 1906 Pure Food and Drug Act required that medicine labels state the quantity of each drug and that drugs meet official standards of purity. Subsequent public service campaigns urging people not to use patent medicines containing opiates probably reduced the number of people becoming addicted to these drugs; there was a modest decline in opiate addiction from the peak in the 1890s until 1914 (Brecher 1972). Yet there were still no national laws concerning opiates or cocaine. Restrictions on their availability would emerge from growing concern, legal ingenuity, and the unexpected involvement of the federal government with the international trade in narcotics (Musto 1999).

The Harrison Narcotic Act of 1914

In 1914, the landmark federal Harrison Narcotic Act was passed. The act required a strict accounting of opium and coca and their derivatives from their point of entry into the United States to their dispensing to a patient. To accomplish this, the act called for a small tax at each transfer and required permits from the Treasury Department for each transaction. Patients were exempt from the tax and the need for a permit (Musto 1991). The law applied to manufacturers, importers, pharmacists, and physicians prescribing narcotics, although patent-medicine manufacturers were exempted providing that they limited the quantities of opium, morphine, or heroin in each preparation. At its face value, the Harrison Narcotic Act was merely a law for the orderly marketing of opium, morphine, heroin, and other drugs, and the right of a physician to prescribe these drugs appeared unambiguous: "Nothing contained in this section shall apply . . . to the dispensing or distribution of any of the aforesaid drugs to a patient by a physician, dentist, or veterinary surgeon registered under this Act in the course of his professional practice only" (Brecher 1972). Registered physicians were required only to keep records of drugs dispensed or prescribed. It is unlikely that a single legislator realized in 1914 that the Harrison Narcotic Act would ultimately be deemed a prohibition law (Casey 1978). By July 1916, 124,000 physicians, 47,000 retail pharmacists, 37,000 dentists, 11,000 veterinarians, and 1,600 manufacturers, importers, and wholesalers had registered (Musto 1999).

From the 1880s to the period following World War I, opinion both outside and inside the medical profession increasingly held physicians largely responsible for the serious opiate addiction problems sweeping the United States (Manchikanti, Brown, and Singh 2002). Following the passage of the Harrison Act, law enforcement interpreted the clause "in the course of his professional practice only" as banning doctors from prescribing opiates to their addicted patients to maintain them on opiates without a medical reason, and addiction was not considered a disease state (Casey 1978). The reasoning was that since addiction was not a disease, an addict was not a patient, and opiates dispensed to or prescribed for them by a physician were therefore being supplied outside the limits of professional practice. This view transformed a law intended to ensure the orderly marketing of narcotics into a law prohibiting the dispensing of narcotics to addicts by a physician's prescription (Casey 1978).

Many physicians were arrested under this interpretation, and some were convicted and imprisoned. Even those who escaped conviction suffered career devastation by the publicity surrounding their prosecution. The medical profession quickly learned that to supply opiates to addicts was to court disaster (Brecher 1972), and by the end of the 1920s, these heavy-handed tactics had taken their toll on physicians who became very fearful of prescribing narcotics (Manchikanti, Brown, and Singh 2002).

For all practical purposes, opium and cocaine could no longer be obtained legally, and new illicit channels filled the void to accommodate the demand among drug users. The use of opiates actually continued at roughly the same level as before the passage of the Harrison Act (Casey 1978).

When the Supreme Court ruled in the early 1920s that prescribing for addictions was not legitimate medical practice, the interpretation made addiction a federal crime. These series of court rulings drove addicts into urban centers for access to the illicit supply and forced formerly decent and responsible citizens who had acquired an opiate addiction to engage in criminal conduct. By 1923, as many as 75% of women in the federal prison system were Harrison Act prisoners (Clark 1976; Casey 1978).

In 1918, just four years after the passage of the Harrison Act, a study by Congress arrived at the following conclusions:

- Opiates and cocaine were being used by about a million people.
- The "underground" traffic in narcotic drugs was comparable to the legitimate medical traffic.
- Drug dealers and traffickers were organized on a national level and were smuggling the drugs through seaports and across the Canadian or Mexican borders (Casey 1978).
- The wrongful use of narcotic drugs had increased since passage of the Harrison Act in two major cities (Brecher 1972).

As a result of those findings, Congress strengthened the Harrison Act. In 1924, a law prohibiting the importation of heroin for any purpose, including medical use, was enacted (Casey 1978). However, the 1924 ban on heroin did not deter the conversion of morphine addicts to heroin. Instead, heroin almost universally replaced morphine after the law was passed (Brecher 1972). Nevertheless, during the 1920s and 1930s morphine and heroin use declined in the United States, with much of the problem confined to the periphery of society and the outcasts of urban areas (Musto 1991).

The severity of federal laws concerning the sale and possession of opiates and cocaine gradually increased following the Harrison Act, culminating in 1956 when the death penalty was introduced as a sentencing option for anyone older than 18 providing heroin to anyone younger than 18 (nobody was executed under this statute). At the same time, mandatory minimum prison sentences were extended to ten years (Musto 1991).

The Controlled Substances Act of 1970

The Controlled Substances Act (CSA), which is Title II and Title III of the Comprehensive Drug Abuse Prevention and Control Act of 1970, is currently the legal foundation of the U.S. government's stance against drug abuse. This law is a consolidation of numerous laws regulating the manufacture and distribution of narcotics, stimulants, depressants, hallucinogens, and anabolic steroids, as well as precursor chemicals used in their production (DEA 2005). The CSA established a system classifying drugs with a potential for abuse into five schedules determined by their medicinal value, potential for abuse, and safety or dependence liability. All scheduled drugs except those in schedule I are legally available to the public with a prescription (USGAO 2003).

The determining factor for placement of a drug in the CSA system is abuse potential. Although the term "potential for abuse" was not defined in the CSA, the following criteria were used to define the abuse liability of the substance (DEA 2005):

1. Evidence that individuals were taking the substance in amounts sufficient to create personal or community hazard; or

2. Significant diversion of the substance from legitimate drug channels; or

3. Individuals are taking the substance on their own initiative rather than under legitimate medical supervision; or

4. The drug is a new drug with a mechanism of action similar enough to a drug already known to have abuse potential so as to make it reasonable to assume that there may be significant diversion, nonmedical use, individual health hazard, or community safety hazard.

The factors below are considered in determining in which of the five schedules to place a substance following the identification of its abuse potential, or whether a previously scheduled substance needs to be reassigned to a different schedule, (DEA 2005):

1. The drug's actual or relative potential for abuse

2. Scientific evidence of the drug's pharmacological effects

3. The state of current scientific knowledge regarding the substance

4. History and current pattern of abuse of the substance

5. The scope, duration, and significance of abuse

6. The potential risk to the public health

7. The drug's psychic or physiological dependence liability

8. Whether the substance is an immediate precursor of a substance already controlled

After considering these factors, the drug or substance is placed in the most appropriate schedule established by the CSA, defined as follows (DEA 2005):

SCHEDULE I

➤ The substance has a high abuse potential.

➤ The substance has no currently accepted medical use in the United States.

➤ There is a lack of accepted safety for use of the substance under medical supervision.

. . . .

Schedule I substances include heroin, lysergic acid diethylamide (LSD), marijuana, and methaqualone.

SCHEDULE II

➤ The substance has a high abuse potential.

➤ The substance has a currently accepted medical use in the United States.

➤ Abuse of the substance may lead to severe psychological or physical dependence.

. . . .

Schedule II substances include morphine, phencyclidine (PCP), cocaine, methadone, and methamphetamine.

SCHEDULE III

➤ The substance has less abuse potential than the drugs or other substances in schedules I and II.

➤ The substance has a currently accepted medical use in the United States.

➤ Abuse of the substance may lead to moderate or low physical dependence or high psychological dependence.

. . . .

Anabolic steroids, codeine and hydrocodone with aspirin or Tylenol, and certain barbiturates are examples of schedule III substances.

SCHEDULE IV

➤ The substance has a low abuse potential relative to the drugs or other substances in schedule III.

➤ The drug has a currently accepted medical use in the United States.

➤ Abuse of the drug may lead to limited physical dependence or psychological dependence relative to the drugs in schedule III.

. . . .

Drugs in schedule IV include Darvon, Talwin, Equanil, Valium, and Xanax.

SCHEDULE V

➤ The drug has a low abuse potential relative to the drugs in schedule IV.

➤ The drug has a currently accepted medical use in the United States.

➤ Abuse of the drug may lead to limited physical dependence or psychological dependence relative to the drugs or other substances in schedule IV.

. . . .

Cough medicines with codeine are an example of schedule V drugs.

The 1970 CSA was part of an omnibus reform package designed to rationalize, and in some respects to liberalize, U.S. drug policy. While the legislation provided additional resources for law enforcement and a systematic way to regulate the use of most psychoactive drugs, it also abolished mandatory minimum sentences and provided more funding and support for treatment and research. Over the next three decades, Congress continuously amended the act to create a more punitive system of drug control that ultimately characterized the U.S. government's "war on drugs," and by the 1980s, the flexibility and innovative spirit of the original Controlled Substances Act (and the general approach of Nixon-era drug policy) had largely disappeared from American drug policy (Courtwright 2004).

The mid-1980s witnessed the reemergence of harsh and severe drug laws. In 1986, Congress passed the Anti-Drug Abuse Act, which reestablished mandatory minimum sentences, and a similarly named act in 1988, which introduced the death penalty for major traffickers in certain circumstances (Musto 1999).

U.S. Drug Policies and Race

Americans quickly associated smoking opium with Chinese immigrants who arrived after the Civil War to work on railroad construction. This association was one of the earliest examples of a powerful theme in the United States, suggesting a link between a drug and a feared or rejected group within society. Cocaine would be similarly linked with blacks, and marijuana with Latinos, in the twentieth century (Musto 1991).

Researchers have observed that narcotic experts, during periods of the emergence and growing recognition of drug problems in the United States, linked addiction with race. Medical historian David F. Musto notes that "the Southerner's fear of the Negro and the Westerner's fear of the Chinese" shaped American responses to a growing "drug problem" (1987). David T. Courtwright stated that changes in the demographics of the addict population, including race, played a large role in the passage of the Harrison Narcotic Act. Likewise, scholars of race relations in the United States have found frequent references to opium use in anti-Chinese diatribes (1982).

These explanations of narcotic addiction often went beyond associating opium smoking with the Chinese and suggested that the threat posed by opium addiction was merely the "condition" of the Chinese. This use of race as a metaphor for addiction helped shift the conversation of addiction away from the description of behavior and moved it instead to the investigation of essences. Narcotic addiction experts, who often argued that to be an addict was to be *like* the Chinese, further implied that to be Chinese was to be *like* an addict (Morgan 1974).

Although the Chinese introduced opium smoking to the United States in the early 1870s, the connection between opium and the Chinese continued well into the 1900s as part of the drive for laws prohibiting opium (White 1979). Most of the new "addicts," who had become steadily more visible after 1870, were not Chinese and were not opium smokers (Courtwright 1982), but instead used morphine, cocaine, or heroin, with many becoming "addicted" through the care of physicians who sought to treat any number of maladies by the hypodermic injection of opiate drugs. Despite the presence of new drugs and new users, the association of Asians with opiate addiction and its effects persisted into the turn-of-the-century debate surrounding narcotic addiction (Hickman 2000).

The association of particular drugs with marginalized minority groups and foreign enemies has a long history in the United States. The association of opium with the Chinese, cocaine with blacks, alcohol with urban Catholic immigrants, heroin with urban immigrants, marijuana with Latinos, the claim that numerous and diverse foreign enemies were using these drugs against the United States, and the image of drug-crazed bohemians were all integral to the propaganda that generated prohibitionist policies against each of these drugs (White 1979).

Despite the prevalence of addiction in the late nineteenth century, drug addiction was largely viewed as a health problem. Public attitudes about drug use began to change as perceptions about drug users shifted. Opposition to opium smoking grew as it was increasingly linked to Chinese immigrants in the western United States. Reports that the upper classes were taking up opium smoking in New York and other cities led to heightened alarm. Fears that respectable white women were being seduced into a life of prostitution and debauchery in opium dens were inflamed by vivid reports.

In 1902, the Committee on the Acquirement of the Drug Habit of the American Pharmaceutical Association declared: "If the 'Chinaman' cannot get along without his 'dope,' we can get along without him." In 1909, the U.S. international war on drugs began when California prohibited the importation of smokeable opium (Hickman 2000).

Black, Latino, Native American, and many Asian youth were portrayed as violence-prone, traffickers of drugs, and a threat to society. Criminality and deviance were racialized. Surveillance focused on communities of color, immigrants, the unemployed, the undereducated, and the homeless, who continue to be the principal targets of law enforcement efforts to fight the war on drugs (Hickman 2000).

The prominent addiction historian William L. White writes that the beliefs and attitudes generated by the prohibitionist movements of the late nineteenth and early twentieth centuries continue to shape current strategies on use and abuse of mood-altering drugs, and effectively block any attempt to change an outmoded and nonfunctional social policy. The integration of these beliefs into our culture has been so complete that questioning them may be seen as an attack on the broader culture and the institutions that generated these beliefs, such as our national leaders, the law, educational and religious institutions, and the family. What this means is that we must expose and modify the irrational fears and beliefs that have driven current drug policy before we can develop enlightened and rational national drug policies (1979).

White (1979) has also identified several themes in drug prohibition movements:

1. The drug is associated with a hated subgroup of society or a foreign enemy.

2. The drug is identified as the sole cause of many social problems such as crime, violence, and insanity.

3. The survival of the culture is pictured as being dependent on the prohibition of the drug.

4. The concept of controlled or moderate use of the drug is destroyed and replaced by the concept of a "domino theory" of chemical progression.

5. The drug is associated with the corruption of young children, particularly their sexual corruption.

6. Both the user and supplier of the drug are defined as fiends always in search of new victims, and usage of the drug is considered "contagious."

7. Policy options are presented in the dichotomy of either total prohibition or total access.

8. Anyone questioning these assumptions is viciously attacked and characterized as part of the problem that needs to be eliminated.

Changing Viewpoints of Opiate Addiction

The central concept of nineteenth-century medicine as it related to addiction was the concept of *inebriety*. Inebriety was viewed as a disease with different manifestations according to clinical subpopulation and drug choice, such as alcohol inebriety, cocaine inebriety, and morphine inebriety. The disease of inebriety was also thought to stem from multiple pathways, capable of unfolding in diverse patterns, with a variable course and outcome. Inebriety specialists began speaking of the importance of tailoring treatment to disease specifics as early as the 1880s (White 2009).

Most thought not only that drug-dependent individuals used their drug to relieve the symptoms of illness and for the beneficial effects produced by the painkillers and stimulants but also that they needed the drug to maintain a sense of well-being and to feel normal. In the absence of the drug, these dependent users suffered prolonged anxiety, restlessness, sleep disturbance, and other symptoms of drug withdrawal (White 2009). Opioids were used to treat both physical pain and psychiatric illness in an era devoid of psychiatric medications.

The following excerpts were written by prominent addiction experts of the era:

> Opium addiction is a disease, a well-marked functional neurosis, and in
>
> most cases, the vice theory of its origin is incorrect, and the term "opium

habit" a misnomer as it implies, incorrectly so, that the opium using is under the control of the individual. Two causative factors, necessity and desire, exist, but the result is the same—a condition of disease, as evidenced by various functional ills.

(MATTISON 1885)

It is now a matter of established record and proof that narcotic drug addiction is fundamentally a physical disease condition presenting definite and constant clinical symptoms and signs and invariable and characteristic physical phenomena, and that it has associated with it, and especially with its unskillful handling, some of the most agonizing suffering known to humanity.

No theory of drug addiction based on inherent mental degeneracy or deterioration, no exposition or explanation of circumstances, situations or conditions, associated with or incidental to narcotic drug addiction can any longer, in the light of easily available and easily corroborated testimony or record and competent authority, be regarded as worthy of any consideration which ignores or does not completely take into account the established facts and the physical sufferings of narcotic drug addiction—disease.

The worst evils of the narcotic situation are not, as is widely taught, rooted in the inherent depravity and moral weakness of those addicted. They find their origin in opportunity, created by ignorance and neglect and fear, for commercial and other exploitation of the physical suffering resulting from denial of narcotic drug to one addicted.

The worst evil of the narcotic situation in the past few years, and especially since the enforcement of restrictive legislation without provisions for education and adequate treatment, is the rapid increase and spread of criminal and underworld and illicit traffic in narcotic drugs. This exists because conditions have been created which make smuggling and street peddling and criminal and illicit traffic tremendously profitable, and it would not exist otherwise. It is simply and plainly the exploitation of human suffering by the supplying to desperate and diseased individuals at any price which may be demanded, one of the necessities of their immediate existence.

(BISHOP 1919)

The Keeley Cure

The Keeley Institute was an organization founded in 1879 for the treatment of opiate and alcohol addiction by Leslie Keeley, a Civil War surgeon who announced his cure in 1879 with his famed slogan, "Drunkenness is a disease and I can cure it," and his "secret" injections of gold chloride, known as the "Gold Cure." Keeley's cure was allegedly made from "double chloride of gold," but was actually comprised of atropine, strychnine, arsenic, cinchona, and glycerin. Patients at his institutes were gradually weaned from their habits, received periodic injections, and ingested a dram of the formula every two hours, and were also required to follow a regimen of healthful diet, fresh air, exercise, and adequate sleep. Patients were required to pay $160 up front and stay for thirty-one days. It is unknown how many of the 400,000 Keeley graduates remained abstinent from opiates or alcohol (Blair Historic Preservation Alliance; *Time Magazine* 1939). Also unknown are what percentage died of his "cure."

Through his practice, Dr. Keeley eventually amassed a fortune of more than $1 million. However, by 1900 the approach was largely discredited. The Keeley Cure, however, did have some initial success. At one time more than 200 Keely Institute treatment centers existed. Patients who recovered from their addiction were honored as "graduates" and urged to promote the treatment that had helped them. Patients were also encouraged to involve themselves in what would now be referred to as group therapy, a factor that likely contributed to the success of those who remained abstinent. Despite the view that Keeley's "Gold Cure" was merely a successful example of nineteenth-century quackery, Dr. Keeley made an important contribution to the field of addiction treatment as one of the first to widely treat addiction as a medical problem (Blair Historic Preservation Alliance; Nebraska State Historical Society 2005).

Narcotic Clinics, 1912–1925

Among the very first treatment approaches for opiate dependency in the late nineteenth century was controlled dosages of some form of the addictive drug itself. Referred to as "maintenance treatment," this approach aimed to achieve permanent abstinence from illicit opiates by transferring the dependency to a more readily controlled dosage and safer form. Other goals of maintenance therapy included reducing criminal behavior and health risk. Although many U.S. practitioners (out of a humane motive) quietly provided these drugs to their patients as needed, others—referred to as "dope doctors" and regularly vilified in the press—exploited patient dependency to reap enormous profit, which served to discredit this approach. (These were not unlike the "pill mills" of our current era.) Nevertheless, between 1914 and 1924, morphine maintenance programs were established in many cities in the United States; in New York City, more than 7,000 patients were dispensed opiate drugs under the auspices of the city's Department of Health (Drucker 2000).

The general public's reaction to the maintenance approach was negative, and soon, American medicine sought to distance the profession from narcotic maintenance and from the problem of addiction entirely. In 1910, the American Medical Association (still in its infancy) described the provision of drugs to the addict as "immoral" and declared that addiction was outside of its responsibility. Accordingly, the 1914 Harrison Act was interpreted as banning the medical prescription of opiates as addiction treatment. This view, although challenged by concerned practitioners, was upheld in the U.S. Supreme Court throughout the 1920s and had the effect of outlawing maintenance as a medical practice and shutting down the still young and inexperienced drug maintenance treatment programs that had begun to emerge (Drucker 2000). Such a negative view of addicts undermined medical treatment of addiction and distanced the medical profession from people who had this disease.

The first narcotic clinic was opened in 1912 in Jacksonville, Florida, and provided both opiates and cocaine to men and women, blacks and whites. Other clinics followed, particularly after the Treasury Department, in enforcement of the 1914 Harrison Act, prosecuted or threatened with prosecution health professionals who provided maintenance therapy to addicts. A series of clinics in New England were established at the suggestion of officials at the Internal Revenue Bureau. Registration of addicts was permitted so physicians would restrict maintenance to those already addicted. In New York City, the Health Department did not wish to provide opiates, morphine, and heroin on an indefinite basis but did open a clinic at the city Health Department headquarters. This clinic provided heroin, but only as an inducement to registration and eventual detoxification and rehabilitation. Around 7,500 addicts registered, received their drug of choice in dosages gradually decreased until uncomfortably small—usually three to eight grains of morphine daily—and were offered "curative" treatment (see page 49). Most declined to be cured, and of those who opted, an estimated 95% returned to their opiate of choice, which they obtained from the street or a physician (Musto 1999).

In 1919, the Supreme Court made two decisions that greatly affected addicts and their medical treatment: The Supreme Court ruled that the Harrison Act was constitutional and that doctors who maintained addicts were in violation of the Harrison Act. In the first case, the Supreme Court reversed an earlier district court decision dismissing an indictment against a Dr. Doremus of San Antonio, Texas, who had been arrested in 1915 for providing a large supply of morphine to a known addict. On appealing the arrest, the district court decided that the Harrison Act as a revenue measure could not restrict the medical practice of Dr. Doremus. The federal government pursued the case to the Supreme Court, which reversed the district court's decision (Waldorf et al. 1974).

In the second decision, the appeal of a Dr. Webb of a Harrison Act indictment was denied because he had supplied morphine to an addict with the intention of maintaining his opiate use. This decision established that maintenance treatment was against the law unless it was part of a cure. In the event that a doctor could not successfully treat an illness or disease, doctors felt justified in relieving the accompanying pain and suffering. For the addict, the relief was opiates (Waldorf et al. 1974).

These two decisions had an immediate effect. Federal agents of the Narcotics Bureau of the Internal Revenue Service rapidly began indicting doctors in various cities throughout the United States who were known to cater to and prescribe opiates to large numbers of addicts. One month after the decision, federal agents in New York City arrested six physicians, four druggists, and 200 addicts for violation of the Harrison Act on the basis that addicts can not be maintained on opiates (Waldorf et al. 1974).

The decisions and the arrests that followed created panic among many doctors because the regular prescription of opiates to a small number of patients was very common. Many of these patients also suffered from chronic or terminal illness and were being treated in good faith (Waldorf et al. 1974).

The solution to the emergencies created by these laws was to establish clinics or dispensaries to treat and "cure" addicts. Some sprang up spontaneously while others seem to have been established at the instigation of federal agents who anticipated trouble from addicts and doctors when legal supplies of opiates were cut off. At the same time, since World War I had ended the previous year, there was the anticipation of a steady stream of returning soldiers who became addicted in the course of treatment for war injuries. This had been the case after both the Civil and Spanish-American wars, and there was no reason to expect that soldiers from World War I would be different (Waldorf et al. 1974).

The initial objective of narcotic clinics was to stabilize addicts on maintenance opiate medication. However, maintenance was only one objective of the morphine clinics, and not necessarily the primary one, because many addicts suffered from a wide range of illnesses including rheumatism and arthritis, respiratory conditions, and venereal diseases, which were treated by the clinics. Many patients fell into the category of being ill as well as addicted, and detoxification was not attempted until the medical illness was treated. All patients, unless chronically ill or very old, were expected to undergo detoxification and were dropped from the clinic if they resisted. In smaller cities addicts who were dropped usually had to move to another city because they could and would be arrested by the clinic's inspectors; it was still an offense to be an addict (Waldorf et al. 1974).

Beginning in 1919, the Treasury Department started closing the clinics and prosecuting the dispensing physicians and druggists. Their argument was that maintenance treatment interfered with curing addicts of their opiate addiction, and that permitting maintenance clinics to operate contradicted the Treasury Department's position when it indicted and prosecuted physicians and pharmacists for dispensing opiate drugs. Gradually the clinics were closed, the last one in 1925 in Knoxville, Tennessee (Musto 1999).

Detoxification and "The Cure"

Detoxification, referred to as "treatment" and "the cure" by the staff of morphine clinics, became a required program component. During the summer of 1919, the Federal Bureau of Narcotics declared that addiction was curable and that it should be done in hospitals and not outpatient clinics. The technique entailed initial dosage reduction in the morphine clinic, after which the patient was hospitalized and given substitute drugs, typically oral opiates with sedatives, which were reduced over a four- or five-day period. Upon entering treatment, patients were required to sign an agreement stipulating that if they could not endure the withdrawal process in the hospital, the staff could place them in jail during the dose reduction. Although the threat of incarceration was often used, patients were actually seldom jailed. Patients were expected to remain in treatment for at least two weeks, and sometimes as long as a month. Detoxification occurred during the first week. The procedure worked very well; most patients expected the process to be more difficult and protracted than it actually was. The remainder of the time was spent in convalescence. Following detoxification, there was little, if any, follow-up (Waldorf et al. 1974).

At the peak of the maintenance clinics, the number of addicts registered under New York State law numbered about 13,000 in 1920. The demise of the clinics left drug dealers and individual members of the health professions as the focal points of federal prosecution. Most physicians did not want to treat addicts and did not sympathize with their condition. Those physicians who did continue to treat addicts with maintenance doses were threatened and arrested, unless the maintenance had been approved by the local narcotic agent. A great amount of fear accompanied a physician's decision to prescribe opiates to a patient, and with the banning of prescribing opiates to manage addiction, physicians had no effective means to treat opiate addiction (Musto 1999).

From the mid-1930s until the mid-1960s, the entire federal drug treatment system consisted of two prison-hospitals: Fort Worth, Texas, and Lexington, Kentucky, both of which treated federal prisoners. Although the patients/prisoners usually relapsed when they returned to their old environments, the programs and contributions of these two facilities are recognized as laying important groundwork in understanding and treating addiction (Maddux 1978).

The wisdom of forty years of apparently self-defeating police solutions to the drug problem began being questioned by such critics as the sociologist Alfred Lindesmith. A negative utilitarian, he believed that if a law produced many costs and few benefits, it was irrational and should be modified or abolished. This belief was the premise of his influential 1965 study *The Addict and the Law.* In this study, he argued that American addicts were both more numerous and more "impoverished, degraded, and demoralized" than elsewhere in the Western world, and he cited police estimates that up to 50% of big-city crime was committed by addicts to support their addiction (Lindesmith 1965). By contrast, the British system of medical maintenance had resulted in neither serious crime nor an inordinate amount of addiction. Lindesmith and others essentially charged the Narcotics Bureau with benighted prohibitionism, resulting in huge costs to both users and society. "The American narcotics problem," summed up Marie Nyswander, co-originator of methadone maintenance for heroin addiction, in 1965, "is an artificial tragedy with real victims" (Hentoff 1965; Courtwright 2001).

Methadone Maintenance

The wisdom of outlawing maintenance treatment of opiate addicts began to be questioned as early as the mid-1950s by such prominent groups as the American Bar Association. An investigation of the feasibility of maintenance was launched, and the outcome, entitled *Narcotic Drugs: Interim Report of the Joint Committee of the American Bar Association and the American Medical Association on Narcotic Drugs (JCABA and AMAND)* (1958), was authored by a panel of physicians, lawyers, and judges and was based on three years of research in the United States and Britain. The *Interim Report* was a rational and temperate critique of the police approach, with suggestions for further research and trial programs. Casting doubt on "whether drug addicts can be deterred from using drugs by threats of jail or prison sentences," the report recommended the establishment of an experimental outpatient clinic that might, under certain circumstances, provide addicts with opiate drugs so they would stop obtaining the drugs illegally (JCABA and AMAND 1961; Courtwright 2001; Joseph, Stancliff, and Langrod 2000).

Methadone maintenance began as a research project at the Rockefeller University in 1964 and was funded through the Health Research Council (HRC) of New York City in response to the swelling number of heroin addicts in the city following World War II (Joseph, Stancliff, and Langrod 2000).

Six male heroin addicts voluntarily enrolled in the pilot study in 1964. Initially, morphine was used as the maintenance opiate, but proved unsatisfactory since morphine had to be injected several times a day in increasing amounts as tolerance developed. On morphine maintenance, the patients were apathetic, sedated, and preoccupied with receiving the next injection to avoid withdrawal symptoms. Later, methadone was investigated as an alternative to the shortcomings of the shorter-acting opioids. The researchers found that when the patients were maintained on methadone after the point of tolerance to the opiate effects, they were no longer sedated or preoccupied with drugs, their affect was clear, their behavior changed, and many began to plan for employment and school. And perhaps most important, their drug cravings diminished. The six patients ultimately achieved gainful employment while they were maintained on methadone doses of 100–180 mg/d (Joseph, Stancliff, and Langrod 2000). Dole and Nyswander published the seminal paper "A Medical Treatment for Diacetylmorphine (Heroin) Addiction" in 1965, describing methadone maintenance.

Further studies were performed to determine whether methadone would prevent relapse to heroin addiction or respiratory depression if heroin use was resumed. An effective blockade of the reinforcing effects of heroin, morphine, dilaudid, and methadone itself was achieved at 80–120 mg/d or higher (Joseph, Stancliff, and Langrod 2000). In 1966, the clinic model was adopted for expanding methadone maintenance treatment throughout the United States, and positive results in terms of decreased drug use, decreased crime, and safety were reported (Dole and Nyswander 1965; Gerstein and Harwood 1990). By 1969, there were several thousand patients in methadone maintenance treatment in the United States (Rettig and Yarmolinsky 1995). As of February 2009, roughly 1,200 methadone maintenance programs were operating nationwide (USGAO 2009).

Controversies Surrounding Methadone Maintenance

Although the United States was the pioneer in developing and implementing methadone maintenance treatment, old attitudes hostile to maintenance approaches were never totally abandoned and soon began to reassert themselves with methadone as the target. The United States was also the birthplace and remains the spiritual center and home of the worldwide movement of the Twelve Step programs of Alcoholics Anonymous and Narcotics Anonymous, and the drug-free therapeutic communities (TCs) such as Synanon and Phoenix House. Unlike the method prescribed by methadone maintenance, total abstinence from all mood-altering drugs was the principal goal of the Twelve Step and TC programs and constitutes the only acceptable terms for drug users' participation. The contrast between these two treatment philosophies led to a sharp division (Drucker 2000).

Additionally, problems associated with methadone were recognized and reported, sometimes in sensationalistic media reports that contributed to negative attitudes about methadone maintenance. These reports included methadone diversion and methadone overdoses, patients selling their take-home methadone, the excessive prescribing practices of rogue physicians, patients receiving prescriptions for methadone who were not truly opiate-dependent, methadone maintenance patients addicted to other substances, and stories about children overdosing on their parents' take-home methadone. Many of the reports were accurate and the issues involved still exist, but some were exaggerations, a phenomenon which also continues. Criticism came from "drug-free" providers and advocates who viewed methadone maintenance as merely another form of addiction; most law enforcement agencies were skeptical or outright hostile; and some minority groups labeled methadone maintenance "genocide" (Jaffe 1975; Courtwright 1992).

Although the successful methadone patient generally went unnoticed, the worst cases were all too evident around their overly large and often conspicuous clinics in the midst of some of the most embattled communities in the United States. Methadone treatment was commonly and publicly held in contempt, and an urban folklore of methadone's evil qualities soon became conventional wisdom in the drug treatment world. The quality of methadone treatment suffered, reflected in the steady lowering of dosages below therapeutically recommended levels and in the increasingly punitive and controlling character of many methadone maintenance programs. The crack cocaine epidemic of the mid- to late 1980s resulted in opiate addicts who also became addicted to crack. This new group of particularly difficult-to-treat drug users also served to reinforce the strong attitudes already opposed to the use of methadone and further diverted attention from the treatment needs of the much older cohort of heroin addicts. The once rapid expansion of methadone maintenance programs in the United States ground to a halt, stagnation followed, and there has been little growth or innovation of methadone treatment in the United States since the 1970s (Drucker 2000).

A little-known fact is that one of the physicians credited with developing and implementing methadone as a treatment for opiate addiction, Dr. Vincent Dole, was on the General Services Board of Alcoholics Anonymous (AA) and was a friend of AA co-founder Bill Wilson. Wilson had a great deal of respect for Dole's development of methadone treatment for heroin addiction and was not opposed to the use of effective medications such as methadone to treat addicts. Wilson realized that many alcoholics did not respond to AA, dropped out, or never entered the program only to disintegrate or die from the disease, and he eventually asked Dr. Dole to create a drug to treat alcoholism. This encouraged Dole toward the end of his career to conduct alcoholism studies in his laboratory. However, he was unable to find an analogue of alcohol that could be used as a medication to treat alcohol addiction (Dole 1991; Joseph and Woods 2006).

The Therapeutic Community Approach

The growth of treatment facilities in the 1960s and 1970s reflected differing views on the nature of drug abuse and addiction and what was required to treat it effectively. Aside from detoxification units—which were intended to provide a transition to a drug-free state, but typically provided only a brief respite from active addiction—four treatment models for opiate addicts emerged: outpatient methadone maintenance programs, drug-free outpatient programs, short-term residential programs using the Twelve Step model, and long-term, drug-free residential programs called therapeutic communities (TCs) (Institute of Medicine 1990).

The approach taken by TC programs reflects the view that drug addicts had social deficits and required social treatment. This social treatment aspect was an organized effort to resocialize the client, with the community as the agent of personal change. TCs evolved from a self-help perspective as a social movement, and since TCs used a social treatment approach, their directors and program staff were comprised of ex-addicts, social activists, and health professionals (Tims, Jainchill, and De Leon 1994).

TCs emphasized structure and hierarchy within the program, the need to isolate the addict from competing influences during treatment, the need for an extended treatment that is phased and intensive, and clear norms for personal responsibility and behavior. Learning, accepting, and internalizing these norms was achieved through a highly structured treatment process that required active participation by the client in a context of confrontation (to address denial, false beliefs, and defense mechanisms), self-help, and affirmation of program expectations. The change process in the TC uses behavioral and social learning principles, and change is viewed from a behavioral orientation (Tims, Jainchill, and De Leon 1994).

Synanon was the archetype of the therapeutic community; it was founded in Ocean Park, California, in 1958 by Charles Dederich. Dederich had been a successful member of Alcoholics Anonymous for a number of years, but left AA to form his own organization, in part because of uneasiness with opioid addicts within AA. Dederich unambiguously touted the authoritarian nature of Synanon, which was designed to re-create an autocratic family environment to keep the clients in line. He also emphasized confrontational group encounters led by a *Synanist,* an experienced Synanon member. These encounters were intended to make the participants come to terms with their feelings, to take personal responsibility, and to learn alternate coping skills other than drugs and alcohol. Once clients could achieve these goals, they would theoretically be equipped to return to the world and lead "straight" lives (Courtwright 2001).

From the start, Synanon was a highly controversial therapeutic community and counseling style, and it remained so throughout its history. Its confrontive counseling style, once called attack therapy, had its believers and its critics both in and out of the traditional mental health community. Dederich believed that an aggressive, hard-hitting confrontational approach was the only way to penetrate the addict's psychological defenses built up over years or decades. And many clients did respond to the approach—clients who had been resistant to years of incarceration and mental-health-system therapy approaches. However, critics viewed the approach as abusive and degrading. Synanon also emphasized self-help and self-reliance, differing somewhat from AA, which stressed mutual help, personal accountability, and reliance on a Higher Power (Shaffer 1995).

Synanon experienced rapid growth in the late 1950s and into the 1970s, and although the organization received financial support and praise from well-known Hollywood actors, detractors became increasingly vocal in their opposition. Many Synanon members had extensive criminal histories as well as severe opioid addiction, creating fear among some citizens and government officials about who was living in their communities. The concept of former addicts treating recently arrived addicts was also at odds with the established belief that only credentialed professionals were qualified to treat addicts (Shaffer 1995).

Eventually, controversies erupted around media-covered lawsuits about Synanon's alleged influence over its residents' marriage arrangements and child-rearing, reports of physical violence, and Synanon's corporate, business, financial, and legal problems. In the early 1980s, Dederich and a smaller group of Synanon residents moved to a wooded setting in northern California, but the ideal of communal living at Synanon gradually dissipated as members left the community (Shaffer 1995). The Synanon model was eventually reproduced in many parts of the country, especially in New York City, by such organizations as Daytop Village and Phoenix House (Batiste and Yablonsky 1971).

Bias and Stigma Remain

U.S. drug policy has shaped and been shaped by our cultural views of addiction, both as moral failing and as disease. We are moving slowly toward a more informed policy, but the "war on drugs," especially supply reduction, still receives more federal attention and money than prevention and treatment efforts, which would decrease demand. We have improved the medical care and treatment of addiction, and through federally funded research, our understanding of addiction as a brain disease has greatly progressed. However, bias and stigma remain in U.S. culture and limit the care and treatment of addiction in the twenty-first century.

CHAPTER 4

The Background and Characteristics of Prescription Opioid Users

Gender, Age, Race, and Other Characteristics

Gender differences in the prescribing patterns for different classes of psychotropic medication have long been known, with women 18 years and older being much more likely to be prescribed opioid analgesics and anti-anxiety drugs (McCabe, Boyd, and Teter 2006). Gender differences have also been found among abusers of prescription opioids. In a study of 3,821 patients admitted to treatment centers who reported past-month prescription opioid abuse, women were more likely than men to use any kind of prescription opioid (29.8% females versus 21.1% males) and abuse a prescription opioid (15.4% females versus 11.1% males). Factors related to prescription opioid abuse among women included problem drinking, age less than 54 years, inhalant use, residence outside of western United States, and history of drug overdose. Factors seen among the male opiate abusers included age less than 34 years, currently living with their children, residence in the South and Midwest, hallucinogen use, and recent depression. Women prescription opioid abusers were less likely to report a pain problem, although they were more likely to report medical problems compared with women who abused other drugs (Green et al. 2009).

Age

A study of high school students found that illicit users of prescription opioids were significantly more likely to be male, be white, have lower grade point averages, and have higher rates of cigarette smoking, alcohol use, marijuana use, other illicit drug use, and problem behaviors (McCabe and Boyd 2005).

Racial and Ethnic Differences

Racial differences in illicit use of prescription drugs among college students have been noted, with past-year illicit use of prescription opioids significantly higher among white college students (8.2%) than among Hispanic (4.4%), African American (3.4%), and Asian (2.5%) students (McCabe, Boyd, and Teter 2006).

Regional Differences

A large proportion of rural opioid users who report being treated for pain also report the nonmedical use of prescription drugs. Similarly, among the nonmedical users, half reported experiencing pain that interfered with their daily lives, suggesting that many rural prescription drug users are being either incorrectly or perhaps inadequately treated for chronic pain (Havens, Walker, and Leukefeld 2008).

Substantial regional differences have been found in opioid prescribing patterns in the United States. A 2000 study found that an average of 64.2 out of every 1,000 prescriptions were written for oral opioids. The proportion of prescriptions for opioid painkillers varied between states, and ranged from less than 20 per 1,000 to more than 100 per 1,000 prescriptions. States with higher proportions of residents age 15–24 and 65 and older had lower rates of prescriptions for all opioid painkillers. Several factors were associated with regions with high numbers of opioid prescriptions, including the number of surgeons per 1,000 residents, the proportion of the population reporting illicit drug use, and the proportion of residents who were female. Factors related to higher prescribing rates for oxycodone included the proportion of the population age 25–34, and the number of surgeons per 1,000 residents. States with established prescription monitoring programs had among the lowest rates of opioid prescriptions (Curtis et al. 2006).

A study examining the extent of and factors related to geographic variation in opioid prescribing for acute, work-related, low back pain found significant differences between states, ranging from 5.7% (Massachusetts) to 52.9% (South Carolina). This large difference was explained by three factors: state household income inequality, the number of physicians per capita, and workers compensation cost containment effort (Webster et al. 2009).

Subgroups of Prescription Opioid Abusers

Green and Butler (2008) evaluated data on prescription substance abusers entering treatment and identified six subgroups of prescription opioid abusers:

- prescribed misusers
- healthy abusers
- poly-prescription opioid abusers who inject
- poly-prescription opioid abusers who snort
- OxyContin plus heroin abusers
- methadone and other opioid abusers

These classes, or groups, were distinct in their prescription opioid abuse practices and preferences, including drug preferences, reporting of pain problems, preferred routes of administration, and economic background.

Differences also exist between people who abuse prescription opioids obtained on the illicit underground market (illegally) and those who obtain their prescription opioids by doctor shopping (legally). In contrast to the group who obtain opioids illegally, women comprised half of the doctor shoppers, and only a minority of doctor shoppers were younger than 35. The doctor shoppers more closely resembled patients who would typically receive prescription opioids—they were generally older and, as a group, the proportions of men and women were more even. Doctor shoppers tended to come from higher-income counties and to take their opioid drugs orally. Doctor shoppers may represent a subgroup of prescription opioid abusers who are less willing to engage in illegal activities (Hall et al. 2008).

A study comparing prescription opioid abuse rates from 2003 to 2006 with data on the rates of unemployment and poverty, population density, high school graduation rate, and proportion of bachelor's degrees has been conducted (Spiller et al. 2009). The study found two strong connections between poverty rate, unemployment rate, and prescription opioid drug rates, with prescription opioid drug use rates increasing with the poverty rate and unemployment rate. These trends were strongly influenced by the rates of hydrocodone and methadone use and less from the rate of oxycodone use.

An Internet survey of 3,639 undergraduate students examining sub-types of drug users found these characteristics:

- The self-medication subtype was characterized by the motivation to use the drug consistent with the prescription drug's main pharmaceutical indication, use of the drug solely via the oral route of administration, and absence of combining the prescription drug with alcohol.
- The recreational subtypes were characterized by recreational motivation, use by both oral and non-oral routes of administration, and co-ingestion of alcohol.
- Mixed subtypes consisted of other combinations of motivation, routes of administration, and co-ingestion.

Approximately 13% of the survey respondents were recreational sub-types, 39% were self-medication subtypes, and 48% mixed subtypes. The rates of substance use and abuse among self-medication subtypes were generally lower than for other subtypes (McCabe et al. 2009).

An examination of deaths in West Virginia from opioid overdose in 2006 found that the majority of overdose deaths were associated with the non-medical use and diversion of opioid analgesics. The prescription histories of the people who died revealed that drug diversion and doctor shopping involved different subpopulations of prescription drug abusers. Those in the group using diverted drugs resemble those traditionally associated with the abuse of street drugs: more than two-thirds were men, half were younger than 35, and most were unmarried or divorced. Also, people who had used diverted drugs were more likely to have used a nonmedical route of admin-istration, to have combined prescription with illicit drugs in their fatal over-dose, and were more likely to have a recognized history of substance abuse.

Those with a history of abusing drugs obtained through legitimate prescriptions were more likely to begin using prescription drugs to moderate the effects of street drugs and as a substitute opioid when street drugs were not available (Hall et al. 2008).

In order to better understand the patterns of prescription opioid use, misuse, and diversion among street drug users, and to study how the illicit drug culture interfaces with the legitimate therapeutic use of prescription opioids (POs), Davis and Johnson (2008) interviewed 586 street drug abusers from New York City. They recognized the lack of information about PO users compared to that of heroin and cocaine users in New York City. They identified several different categories among the participants in their study:

CATEGORY 1

➤ **Current non-use of POs**

The people in this category do not report PO use. Only 10.1% in this study reported no PO use in their lifetimes, although some of these individuals sold POs or other drugs.

CATEGORY 2

➤ **Medical use without diversion**

These respondents reported using POs for legitimate medical reasons only. In this study, 35.9% had medical use without diversion.

CATEGORY 3

➤ **Medical use with some diversion**

People in this category used POs as indicated for legitimate purposes, but sold or diverted a portion of the medication. In this study, 26.3% of respondents were in this category.

CATEGORY 4

➤ Illicit ingestion

People in this category used POs for intoxication. Some (19.6%) used for euphoria without diverting the medications for sale, while others (18.2%) used the medication for euphoria and sold it.

CATEGORY 5

➤ Diversion only

These respondents sold POs without actually using the drugs themselves, and were rare in this group, with only 8 identified out of 586 persons interviewed.

Risk Factors of Abuse/Dependence

Biological, psychological, sociological, and economic factors determine when an individual will start taking opiates (NIH 1997). Substance use begins with the initial exposure to or experimentation with a drug. Historically, alcohol and nicotine are the first drugs with which young people experiment, which usually occurs before the use of marijuana and other drugs. Early age of initial substance use is consistently linked with increased risk for alcohol and other drug-related problems (McCabe, Boyd, and Young 2007).

Identical twin, family, and adoption studies show that vulnerability to drug abuse or dependence may be an inherited condition, with environmental factors also playing a substantial role. The primary risk factor for addiction is genetic history. Research on twins separated at birth and raised in different environments has demonstrated that both inherited and environmental factors play a role in the origin and development of drug abuse. These adoption studies identified two distinct genetic pathways to drug abuse and dependence. The first is a direct effect of substance abuse in a biologic parent. The second pathway is the indirect effect of a biological parent with antisocial personality disorder, which results in both antisocial personality disorder and drug abuse/dependence in the adoptee. Family studies have found a substantially increased risk for substance abuse, alcoholism, antisocial personality, and depression among the first-degree relatives of opioid-dependent patients compared with relatives of controls. The siblings of opioid-dependent patients were also highly susceptible to abuse and dependence following the initial use of illicit opioids. Studies of identical and fraternal twins indicate substantial heritability for substance abuse and dependence, and have found that roughly half the risk of developing opioid abuse or dependence is due to genetic factors (NIH 1997).

Concerning IV use, social environment plays a major role in determining whether a non-injecting drug user will eventually use drugs by the intravenous (IV) route. Non-injection drug users with social networks that consist of IV drug users are at a greater risk of using drugs through injection. Although most non-injecting drug users initially express negative feelings toward using needles, these feelings can be softened and nullified by several factors, including social pressures from affiliation with a group of IV drug users, the lure or appeal of experimenting with injection, the idea that the drug will be more intense or effective when it is injected, and the belief that one needs to use less of the drug to achieve the same high when it is injected (Budman, Serrano, and Butler 2009).

Medical and prescription drug claims data were used by White and colleagues (2009) to identify patients at risk for prescription opioid misuse or abuse. The following factors were linked with an elevated risk of prescription opioid misuse or abuse over a twelve-month period:

- age 18 to 24 years
- male
- having received twelve or more opioid prescriptions
- opioid prescriptions from three or more pharmacies
- early prescription opioid refills
- escalating morphine dosages

- psychiatric outpatient visits, hospital visits, and diagnoses of non-opioid substance abuse
- depression, post-traumatic stress disorder, and hepatitis

Compared to those reporting nonmedical use of prescription analgesics other than OxyContin, nonmedical OxyContin users were more likely to show a pattern of more serious drug abuse: use of multiple drugs, injection of drugs, and higher rates of abuse and dependence. Approximately 83% of nonmedical OxyContin users reported having used illicit drugs or other prescription medications nonmedically before their first nonmedical use of prescription opioids. Even compared to those who reported nonmedical use of other prescription painkillers, nonmedical OxyContin users already had a more significant pattern of drug abuse before they began using prescription painkillers for nonmedical purposes. These results suggest that nonmedical use of OxyContin is rarely the initiating factor leading to the abuse of other drugs (Sees et al. 2005).

Risk Factors in Adolescents under Age 18

Among youths age 12 to 17, populations at particularly high risk of prescription opioid abuse include females, African Americans, those of lower socioeconomic status, and those who have favorable attitudes toward illicit drugs, detached parents, or friends who use illicit drugs. The use of other illicit drugs was the strongest predictor of nonmedical use of prescription opioids for this age group (Sung et al. 2005). An earlier age of the initial nonmedical opioid use is a powerful predictor for the development of prescription drug abuse and dependence (McCabe, Boyd, and Young 2007).

Risk Factors in College Students

A 2003 study of 9,161 undergraduate students found that most who were nonmedical users of prescription drugs obtained the drugs from peers. Students who obtained prescription medication from peers had much higher rates of alcohol and other drug use than students who did not use prescription drugs illicitly and students who obtained prescription medication from family members (McCabe et al. 2005).

Another survey of students from 119 four-year colleges found that nonmedical prescription opioid use was more likely to occur among students who were white, lived in fraternity and sorority houses, attended more competitive colleges, earned lower grade-point averages, and reported higher rates of substance use and other risky behaviors (McCabe et al. 2005).

Young adults who score high on measures of sensation-seeking traits—that is, "thrill seekers"—do not perceive the same risks with drug use as people who score lower in sensation-seeking traits. People with sensation-seeking and thrill-seeking tendencies may actually view drug use risk as attractive instead of something to avoid. Because prescription opioids have been approved for medical use, they are often seen as inherently "safer" than illicit drugs. Both those with a low level of perceived harmfulness of prescription opioids and those high in sensation-seeking traits are at an increased risk of using prescription opioids nonmedically. The effect of high perceived harmfulness protects against the use of street drugs, but not against the nonmedical use of prescription opioids. Thus, increasing the perceived harmfulness of prescription opioids may be a viable prevention strategy for many students, but other approaches might need to be developed to deter high-sensation seekers (Arria et al. 2008).

Risk Factors for Abuse/Dependence in Pain Patients

Chronic pain is highly prevalent in the United States. Approximately 9% of Americans suffer from chronic, non-cancer-related pain (Trescot et al. 2006), and chronic pain affects approximately 50 million Americans every year (Passik 2009). In clinics specializing in pain management, as many as 90% of the patients receive opioids for chronic pain, and opioids are by far the most abused prescription drugs, especially in chronic pain settings (Manchikanti and Singh 2008).

Differences in the subjective response of chronic pain patients treated with opiates for the first time suggest that some patients who develop euphoria, stimulation, and other experiences not typically associated with opioid drugs when they are taken for pain may be at heightened risk for developing prescription opioid addiction (Bieber et al. 2008).

A study examining opioid misuse among patients enrolled in a chronic pain disease management program found that opiate abuse occurred often, with 32% of patients misusing opioids over the course of one year.

The pain patients who abused opioids were more likely to have a history of alcohol or cocaine abuse and alcohol or drug-related problems (Ives et al. 2006).

Motivation for Using Prescription Opioids

The nonmedical use of prescription opioids can be driven by a variety of factors and desires, including (Zacny and Lichtor 2008)

- pain relief
- getting high
- experimentation
- sleep induction
- anxiety relief
- greater perceived safety than street drugs
- to counteract the effects of other drugs
- addiction to the drug

Some motivational factors can overlap, as in the case of the street drug user with physical ailments that require legitimate prescriptions of high-potency opioids. This is more common among older addicts, who are especially likely to have a wide range of conditions involving pain, such as wounds from fights and accidents, diabetes, cancer, intestinal disorders, HIV/AIDS, and arthritis (van Ness, Davis, and Johnson 2004).

Adolescent Users

The motivation to use prescription opioids and other prescription drugs among adolescents was studied by the Partnership for a Drug-Free America. The research (Pasierb 2006) found that teens see distinct benefits from different types of prescription drugs, and that their motivation to use different substances varies according to whether they want to simply get high, to cope with emotional or psychological problems, to change their body, or to perform schoolwork more effectively (Manchikanti 2006).

Teenagers primarily use marijuana as a party drug, with a study finding 81% of teens using it to get high and only 16% using it to deal with problems.

In contrast, a sizable number of teens self-medicated with prescription drugs in order to improve academic performance or to deal with stress or depression. Roughly 43% of teens reported using prescription stimulants like Adderall or Ritalin without a doctor's prescription to help with school-work, 31% said they used stimulants to deal with problems, and 22% said they used stimulants to get high. Nearly 50% indicated they used prescription opioids to get high, and 40% also used them to help cope with problems (Manchikanti 2006).

A study of the motivation for the nonmedical use of prescription opioids among 12,441 high school seniors from 2002 to 2006 found that more than 1 in 10 students reported the nonmedical use of prescription opioids, of these students 45% indicated the relief of physical pain as an important motivation. Among students motivated only by pain relief, the risk of heavy drinking and other drug use was lower than among nonmedical users who used opioids for other reasons. The authors of this study concluded that the motivation for nonmedical prescription opioid use should be considered when working with adolescents who report using prescription opioids (McCabe et al. 2009).

A 2005 survey of students in grades 7–12 found that 12% had used prescription opioids for nonmedical purposes in the past year. A sizable number of these students used opioids for reasons that increased their risk for developing substance abuse problems, including a desire for sleep, for sedation and/or anxiety reduction, and for a stimulant effect (Boyd et al. 2006).

College Students

Among college students, the most frequent reason provided for the non-medical use of prescription opioids was to relieve pain. When this was their sole reason for use, these students were not at an increased risk of other substance abuse problems (McCabe, Boyd, and Young 2007). This study also found that nonmedical users who obtained prescription opioids from their parents were not at the same increased risk for alcohol and other drug problems as students who obtained the drugs from non-parental sources (McCabe, Boyd, and Young 2007).

Among teenage and college-age students, nonmedical users of prescription opioids with motives other than pain relief, who obtain prescription opioids from non-parental sources, and who report non-oral routes of administration are at increased risk for substance abuse problems (McCabe, Boyd, and Young 2007).

Differences between Prescription Opioid Users and Heroin Users

Patients admitted to treatment for addiction to heroin often have different backgrounds than patients who seek treatment for addiction to prescription opioids. Among patients admitted to publicly funded treatment facilities in 2003, 47% of non-heroin opioid users were female compared with 32% of the heroin users. Non-heroin opioid users were more likely than heroin users to be entering treatment for the first time (40% versus 22%), to be Caucasian (89% versus 48%), to have some college education (32% versus 17%), and to be employed full time (23% versus 12%) (SAMHSA 2006a).

A Canadian study found that compared to heroin users only, both people who used only prescription opioids and people who used both prescription opioid and heroin were more likely to be older and use benzodiazepines and cocaine. Also, prescription opioid-only users were more likely to be Caucasian, to have legitimate income, to use drugs by non-injection, to have physical health problems, and to use private physician services (Fischer et al. 2008).

In a study of people seeking treatment that compared prescription opioid-using adolescents with heroin-using adolescents, both groups had high rates of psychiatric disorders (83%) and moderately prominent depression symptoms. The heroin-only teens were more likely to have dropped out of school, be diagnosed as opioid dependent, and inject drugs. The prescription opioid-using teens were more likely to have problems with multiple substances such as prescription sedatives and stimulants, have a current diagnosis of attention deficit/hyperactivity disorder (ADHD), and report selling drugs, and were more likely to be court ordered into treatment and report previous psychiatric treatment (Subramaniam and Stitzer 2009).

Societal and Economic Cost of
Prescription Opioid Abuse

The economic costs of prescription opioid abuse are substantial, both to society and to the payers of medical services, as well as to the users themselves. However, the economic burden is just one part of the larger drug abuse problem in the United States. According to a study prepared for the Office of National Drug Control Policy (ONDCP), the cost of drug abuse in the United States in 2002 was estimated at $180.8 billion (ONDCP 2004). This estimate included resources used to address health and crime consequences, and loss of productivity resulting from disability, death, and withdrawal from the workforce (Strassels 2009).

The economic consequences of prescription opioid abuse and associated problems in the United States are significant. In 2001, the total cost of prescription opioid abuse was estimated at $9.2 billion, including 30% ($2.8 billion) for health care costs, 50% ($4.6 billion) for lost productivity, and 20% ($1.8 billion) for criminal justice. The rise in prescription opiate abuse since these data were collected suggests an increasing economic burden (Birnbaum et al. 2006; Strassels 2009).

In a study examining the direct medical costs of opioid abusers versus nonabusing individuals enrolled in a large health care plan, the average annual health care costs were more than eight times higher for the opioid abusers than for nonabusers ($15,884 versus $1,830, respectively). The high costs for opioid abusers were linked primarily with the high frequency of costly related medical conditions and the high use of medical services and prescription benefits (White et al. 2005).

Loss of work or the inability to work due to physical limitation such as pain persisting longer than ninety days is considered "chronic" and has profound psychosocial consequences that compound patients' suffering. A study evaluated the link between opioid therapy for back pain and chronic work loss using a reference group not receiving prescription opiates. The odds of chronic work loss were six times greater among patients receiving CSA schedule II opiates. The odds of chronic work loss were eleven to fourteen times greater for patients receiving opioid prescriptions of any type for ninety days or more. The study also found that three years following the injury, the health care costs of patients receiving schedule II opioids was $19,453 higher on average than the costs of patients in the reference group. The authors of this study conclude that for many previously employed workers with chronic pain, opioid therapy does not seem to arrest the cycle of work loss and pain (Volinn, Fargo, and Fine 2009).

Supply Factors Contributing to Prescription Opioid Abuse

History has repeatedly shown a direct link between the availability of a drug and the patterns of its abuse, and research by Dasgupta, Jonsson, and Brownstein (2008) and Brownstein and colleagues (2010) suggest a direct relationship between the amount of a prescription opioid dispensed for medical purposes in a given geographic region and its abuse in that region (Budman, Serrano, and Butler 2009). Analysis of the 2006 National Survey of Drug Use and Health indicates that the increase in prescription opioid misuse is connected more with the greater general availability of these medications than misuse by those who were directly prescribed the medications (Denisco, Chandler, and Compton 2008).

The legitimate expansion in the use of prescription painkillers for severe chronic non-malignant pain, in conjunction with the introduction of high-dose extended-release oral tablet formulations of opioids, has also increased the opportunities for the nonmedical use of these prescribed drugs (Woolf and Hashmi 2004).

Both supply and demand factors are fueling the recent explosion in the nonmedical use and abuse of prescription opioids. Supply-side factors related to increased use include the Internet, systemic changes in how pain is managed, individual physician issues, drug diversion, and sharing by friends and family.

Internet Access

Beginning around 1999, Internet pharmacies have provided a convenient alternative for individuals to fill prescriptions (Kraman 2004; Cole 2004; Caywood 2003). In 2003, the U.S. Government Accountability Office

(USGAO) estimated that about 400 Internet pharmacies were selling drugs illegally, with approximately 50% of these pharmacies located outside the United States (USGAO 2000). Rogue sites operating under the guise of legitimacy provide controlled substances to people without prescriptions (Manchikanti 2006). No-prescription websites (NPWs) are online pharmacies that supply consumers with controlled substances without a valid prescription (Gordon, Forman, and Siatkowski 2006).

The National Center on Addiction and Substance Abuse (CASA) at Columbia University has been tracking the availability of controlled prescription drugs over the Internet for several years. Online trafficking of controlled prescription drugs grew rapidly since the first Internet pharmacies began in 1999. The number of websites selling controlled prescription drugs increased between 2004 and 2007, but declined in 2008, possibly due to the effort by federal and state governments, and financial institutions to crack down on Internet trafficking. The DEA reported that in 2006, roughly 11% of prescriptions filled by traditional (brick and mortar) pharmacies were for controlled substances, in contrast to the 95% of prescriptions filled by Internet pharmacies (CASA 2008).

The Pew Internet and American Life Project reported that in 2004, more than 80% of adolescents went online at least monthly, and that 43% of teen and 66% of adult Internet users made purchases over the Internet. Similarly, 79% of adults used the Internet to obtain health and medical information. The global reach, ease of use, and anonymity of the Internet make it as easy for an adolescent to purchase drugs as it is to purchase a CD with a credit card, PayPal, or even cash. Some sites provide drugs free initially without immediate payment (Manchikanti 2006).

A Google or Yahoo search using the term "Vicodin" returned 40% to 50% NPWs in the top 100 sites, with no links to addiction health information websites. Thus, NPWs represent an important development in the sale of illicit drugs because of the ease with which controlled substances can be sold with relative anonymity (Forman, Marlowe, and McLellan 2006). In 2008, benzodiazepines were the controlled prescription drugs most frequently sold over the Internet, followed by opiates. The most frequently offered opioid drugs were hydrocodone (e.g., Vicodin, Lortab), codeine, oxycodone (e.g., Percocet), and propoxyphene (e.g., Darvocet, Darvon)

(CASA 2008). These sites sell mostly schedule III medications to avoid the stricter requirements of schedule II medications.

The accessibility of rogue Internet pharmacies and NPWs raises several concerns among law enforcement and public health officials. These include their ability to evade state licensing requirements and standards, dispense controlled substances without a prescription, and provide fake, substandard, or inappropriate medication (USGAO 2000). However, state and federal laws governing traditional pharmacy stores still apply to Internet sales regardless of the method used by an Internet pharmacy to dispense the medication. The National Center on Addiction and Substance Abuse at Columbia University (2005) has reported the number of Internet pharmacies in operation at any one time has reached as high as 1,400. ComScore reported that 17.4 million people visited an online pharmacy in the fourth quarter of 2004, 14% more than the previous quarter (Manchikanti 2006). Sixty-three percent of these sites did not require a prescription to obtain controlled substances. Thus, sales of psychoactive prescription drugs over the Internet have not only become a major business but also present new challenges to drug abuse prevention and treatment (Falco 2006).

Interestingly, in a study examining the Internet as a source of prescription opioid drugs, 1,116 prescription drug abusers admitted to treatment were asked where they obtained their drugs. Dealers, friends or relatives, and doctors' prescriptions were listed as a source of drugs with equal frequency (approximately 50%–65%), with theft and forgery far behind at 20%. The Internet was mentioned by fewer than 6% of respondents. The authors then attempted to purchase schedule II and III opioids from a random sample of Internet sites and were unsuccessful in purchasing a single scheduled opioid analgesic. They concluded that concerns over the Internet substantially contributing to the diversion of scheduled prescription opioid analgesics may be overstated (Cicero et al. 2008).

Any discussion of the Internet as a facilitator of the nonmedical use of prescription opioids would be incomplete without mentioning its role in providing information on how to use drugs using alternate routes of administration, and how to alter medications designed to prevent abuse, including step-by-step instructions.

Drug tampering is defined as physical or chemical alteration of a specific drug formulation for the purpose of enhancing the drug effect, increasing the rate of onset of the desired drug effect, eliminating the undesired active and inactive constituents, and chemically modifying the active compound. Although the exact figures are unknown, the Internet appears to be a prime source of information for misusers interested in tampering with drug formulations (Cone 2006).

A study by Boyer, Shannon, and Hibberd (2005) found that online information on psychoactive drugs influences a broad range of drug use behaviors, especially among innovative drug users. Additionally, these users alter their drug use and try new behaviors—such as modifying the use of their preferred drugs, stopping or reducing psychoactive substance abuse, and using new drugs and drug combinations—as the result of information located on the Internet. Interestingly, such practices can help drug users minimize the risks associated with drug use—a finding that suggests that online information can actually reduce the harm associated with psychoactive substance abuse. Also, youthful drug abusers seek data from an unexpected breadth of online resources, including federal government antidrug websites, electronic medical textbooks, online vendors of psychoactive agents, web forums, and online drug encyclopedias. However, they seem to prefer websites that promote the use of drugs, such as online drug encyclopedias, typified by Erowid.org. Such a preference may reflect the belief that online encyclopedias contain information that is more truthful and reliable than that contained in government websites (Szalavitz 2001). These findings are important because adolescents readily accept information from the Internet, and younger users may unconsciously append information obtained from the Internet into beliefs and behaviors that are being developed (Shirer). For populations raised on e-mail, instant messaging, and immediate information, seeking data on psychoactive substances from electronic sources (and spontaneous trust of those sources) may be normal behavior (Shirer). The information available on online drug encyclopedias has been linked with adolescent drug abuse and represents a hazard to a population that still needs adult supervision and guidance (Suler 1998; Henretig et al. 1998).

Around 2003, Internet sites began appearing that detailed the recreational use of prescription opiates, even posting recipes on how to heighten the drug's intensity. The traffic on some of the sites is enormous. One, which includes around 3,000 personal accounts of experiences with a wide range of legal and illicit drugs, receives an average of 420,000 hits a day. "Some people post their progress on beating a new formulation almost on a daily basis. Then others respond with questions and experiences of their own—it feeds on itself," says toxicologist Edward Cone (Muir 2006). For instance, some sites discuss how to tamper with skin patches designed to slowly release the opioid painkiller fentanyl. Users sometimes extract the drug from the transdermal patch to eat, inject, or smoke. Yet a single patch can contain enough fentanyl to kill several people, according to toxicologist Bruce Goldberger from the University of Florida in Gainesville. "It's like Russian roulette—you just don't know how much drug you're going to get," he said (Muir 2006).

Systemic Changes in Approach to Pain Management

Pain is the most common reason that people go to the doctor, yet pain is often inadequately treated. Failure to provide relief from pain exacts an enormous social cost from lost productivity, needless suffering, and excessive health care expenditures. Numerous public policy groups and medical organizations, including the American Medical Association (AMA 1990), have issued strong statements attesting that medical practice does not meet acceptable levels of quality when it comes to the diagnosis and management of conditions requiring treatment with a controlled substance, such as pain conditions (Parran 1997; Longo et al. 2000).

The widespread awareness of pain as an undertreated condition and a major health problem in the United States led to the development of initiatives to address the multiple barriers believed to be responsible for the insufficient management of pain (Kentucky All Schedule Prescription Electronic Reporting [KASPER] 2006). Patient advocacy groups and professional organizations were formed, with the objective of improving the management of pain (KASPER 2006). Numerous clinical guidelines were also developed. In addition, based on the influence of the advocacy groups, more than one-third of state legislatures passed intractable pain treatment acts that provided immunity from discipline for physicians who prescribe opioids within the requirements of the statute (Manchikanti 2006).

This focus on more aggressive treatment of pain in the medical field, and the unprecedented demand for proper pain management among patients and advocacy groups led to exponential growth in prescriptions for opiate painkillers. Specific factors contributing to this surge in the prescribing of opiates include (Manchikanti 2006)

- pharmaceutical companies providing marketing and gifts to prescribing physicians
- numerous organizations providing guidelines and standards on pain control
- patient advocacy groups demanding opioids for nonmalignant pain
- enactment of the Patients' Bill of Rights in many states
- regulations mandating the monitoring and appropriate treatment of pain, which were misunderstood by the media and the public
- perceived patient's right to pain relief

Physicians have embraced the concept of long-term opioid treatment for chronic noncancer pain as seen by increased prescribing. This increase in opioid prescriptions for chronic noncancer pain coincides with the significant increase of prescription opioid abuse (Colameco, Coren, and Ciervo 2009). Physician practice and patient expectations have resulted in increased prescriptions of opioids to treat pain. Primary care physicians are expected to address numerous, difficult issues in a matter of minutes while providing a pleasing experience for the patient. Some physicians also have less time for appointments. Prescribing an opioid is pleasing and quick. Patients want rapid pain relief, and initially opioids provide this. It has become commonplace to receive opioid pain medications for all levels of pain, from mild to severe, neglecting other types of treatment, and no longer reserving the opioids for moderate to severe pain.

Individual Physician Factors

Another factor contributing to the increased prescribing of opioids is the increasingly prominent role played by primary care physicians in pain management. Primary care physicians prescribe most of the opioid analgesics in the United States, yet they may be less able to distinguish legitimate pain patients from those trying to manipulate them into prescribing prescription opioids (Inciardi et al. 2009).

Countertransference and Codependence

Countertransference refers to feelings associated with an emotional response of a caregiver to a patient. It is only partially conscious, is always present, and is determined by the physician's own background, emotions, issues, and so on (Longo et al. 2000). *Codependence* is a form of countertransference that may be thought of as the behavioral characteristics of people who are involved in ostensibly helpful relationships with patients who are addicted. The relationship inadvertently results in harm to one or both individuals because the *codependent* is unable to maintain appropriate boundaries or limits in the relationship. A psychological system of denial or identification is created around the relationship, perpetuating it despite the resulting harm. People who are codependent unconsciously fear anger and abandonment if they refuse to gratify the patient's demands, no matter how unreasonable they are (Longo et al. 2000).

An example of codependence is a husband who wakes up hung over after a bout of uncontrolled drinking and asks his wife to call in sick for him at his workplace. In a healthy relationship, the wife will not make the call and will explain that he needs to take responsibility for his own actions. The codependent wife, on the other hand, will compromise her personal integrity and call the employer for her husband (Longo et al. 2000).

Codependence and countertransference may arise from aspects in the physician's background that affect his or her ability to treat patients with drug addictions (Longo et al. 2000).

Physicians who decide to prescribe controlled substances to patients with addictions should be aware that they may be drawn into the patient's denial (Johnson 1998). The physician should pay attention to any unusual emotional responses in himself or herself. These include anger, guilt, a wish to disengage, pity, revulsion, and other emotions different from his or her usual experiences of confidence and empathy in patient interactions (Longo et al. 2000). Physicians are highly susceptible to being drawn into these compromising situations through the process of projective identification, in which patients project their difficulties in such a way that physicians respond without realizing that they are reacting out of emotion, allowing patients to take advantage of them. Patients with addictions are notoriously prone to projecting onto physicians the message that "my problem is now your problem" (Longo et al. 2000).

There is a fine line between empathy and codependence. In physicians, codependence involves overstepping one's boundaries and limits, combined with the fear that the patient will reject him or her if the desired prescription is not delivered. Exactly where the boundaries lie in prescribing controlled substances to patients with addiction is controversial, but learning more about these issues can improve clinical outcomes and risk management (Longo et al. 2000).

Patients who are actively addicted may learn that the physician's enabling instincts and discomfort with confrontation are so great that the physician's initial "no" can be turned into a "yes" if enough pressure is applied. In such situations, a basic clinical survival skill is to mean "no" when saying "no" and to stick with it. The physician may effectively shift discomfort to the patient while still refusing to prescribe by making statements such as "I'm feeling pushed by you to write a prescription today that is not medically indicated and this makes me concerned about you. We need to talk about your use of alcohol [or other substances]" (Longo et al. 2000).

Knowledge and Practice-related Issues

Often, physicians are now aware that many patients seeking pain relief for chronic, nonmalignant pain have underlying psychosocial problems and need psychological or rehabilitation services, or some other type of intervention, not pain medications. In busy medical practices, especially primary care settings, a thorough diagnosis of the origin and type of pain and a comprehensive pain management approach are often difficult to achieve and psychological issues are not considered. As a result, prescription opioids may make up the entire pain management plan and are used for the treatment of psychic pain, not necessarily physical pain. Additionally, aggressive marketing by the pharmaceutical sales force to physicians who prescribe OxyContin and other opioids has contributed to the overprescribing of these medications to patients for whom alternative or nonmedication interventions may have been more appropriate and without the risk of opioids (Manchikanti 2006).

Overprescribing Physicians

The American Medical Association describes four mechanisms—dated, duped, dishonest, and disabled (the four Ds)—by which a physician overprescribes (AMA 1990; Parran 1997; Longo et al. 2000).

Dated refers to physicians whose knowledge of pharmacology and the differential diagnosis and management of chronic pain, anxiety, insomnia, and addiction is outdated and obsolete. Physicians tend to be more out of date in their knowledge and less confident in their skills in these areas than in other areas of medical practice. Often the problem is not one of being outdated, but having never been adequately trained or informed about the proper treatment of pain and/or addiction.

Duped refers to the susceptibility of being misled by the patient. Physicians are generally a caring, trusting group of professionals who are trying to help their patients in an open and honest relationship based on mutual respect, and they may be vulnerable to a manipulative patient. Most physicians count on their patients to provide an accurate, honest medical history. It is the basis of the doctor-patient relationship, but those with addiction are regularly dishonest.

Dishonest physicians are uncommon, but there are corrupt physicians in every geographic area who are willing to write prescriptions for controlled substances in exchange for financial gain or sexual favors.

Disabled physicians are defined in this context as physicians with a medical or psychiatric disability, such as addiction, bipolar disorder, or a personality disorder. These physicians may be careless prescribers of controlled substances and may be less likely to confront patients who are abusing substances out of fear of turning suspicion on themselves.

Illicit Prescribing versus Malprescribing

Although rare, some physicians do write illicit prescriptions in an effort to divert prescription drugs for enormous profits. More common is the malprescribing of controlled substances, which is most often due to knowledge deficits, but can also be due to inappropriate prescribing through "pill mills." Arrests by the DEA of physician prescribers have actually decreased from 81 in 1999 to 63 in 2005, although actions by medical licensure boards have been increasing (Manchikanti 2006).

Diversion

Diversion means rerouting prescription opioids intended for legitimate medical use to the illicit market, or the rerouting from legitimate patients for medical use to people who intend to use them for nonmedical purposes. The diversion of prescription opioids occurs along every point in the drug delivery process, from the original manufacturing site to the wholesale distributor, the physician's office, the retail pharmacy, or the patient (Weathermon 1999). The DEA has estimated that prescription drug diversion is a $25 billion-a-year industry, with opioids probably comprising the majority of this figure (Conlin 1990; USGAO 2003).

Diverting prescription opioids into the illicit market occurs in a number of ways. These include the illegal sale of prescriptions by physicians and pharmacists; "doctor shopping"; theft, forgery, or alteration of prescriptions by health care workers and patients; robberies and thefts from manufacturers, transport companies, distributors, and pharmacies; and thefts of institutional drug supplies. Diversion of substantial amounts of prescription opioids and benzodiazepines also occurs through residential burglaries and cross-border smuggling at both retail and wholesale levels (Inciardi et al. 2007). Additional channels of diversion include "shorting" (undercounting), pilferage, and recycling of medications by pharmacists and pharmacy employees; medicine cabinet thefts by cleaning and repair personnel in residential settings; theft of guests' medications by hotel repair and housekeeping staff; and Medicare, Medicaid, and other insurance fraud by patients, pharmacists, and street dealers (Inciardi et al. 2007). Many pill-abusing teens and young adults obtain their drugs from friends and relatives, through medicine cabinet thefts, medication trading at school, and thefts and robberies of medications from other students (SAMHSA 2007a). As described above, the Internet may also be a significant source for illicit purchases of prescription opioids (CASA 2005; CASA 2007).

The increased diversion of legitimate prescription opioids to illicit use may be attributable to the following (Manchikanti 2006):

- significant increases in drug availability through prescriptions
- exponential growth in retail opioid sales
- the renewed interest and an unprecedented demand for psychotherapeutic drugs
- a 154% increase in opioid prescriptions from 1992 to 2002, compared with a 57% increase of all prescriptions and a 13% population increase during the same period (CASA 2005; Kraman 2004; McCaskill 2002; National Committee Pharmacists Association [NCPA] 1999)
- exponential growth in opioid and other psychotherapeutic drug prescriptions in Medicaid, workers compensation, and managed care populations (KASPER 2006; Mahowald, Singh, and Majeski 2005)
- the number of prescriptions for hydrocodone and oxycodone reaching 120 million in 2005 (Volkow 2006)

Prescription opioids used by adults are typically diverted through doctor shopping, illegal Internet pharmacies, drug theft, prescription forgery, or illicit prescriptions by physicians, while diverted opioids used by youths typically originate by stealing them from relatives or buying them from classmates who are selling legitimate prescriptions (Manchikanti 2006).

Patient Behavior

Patients may exhibit manipulative, demanding behavior to obtain medication. This is referred to as drug-seeking behavior. The patient may imply that the only possible solution to a medical problem is a prescription of a medication with a high abuse potential. For example, the patient may describe symptoms that markedly deviate from objective evidence or the physical examination findings. The patient may insist on receiving a prescription for a controlled substance on the first visit and argue that nonaddictive medications "don't work." The patient may claim to have an allergy to nonaddictive medications or may make remarks about having a high tolerance to drugs, may lose prescriptions, or may run out of prescriptions prematurely (Longo et al. 2000).

The patient may also sell or forge prescriptions or may use the prescriptions of other people, such as family members and friends. Some patients manipulate the situation by pitting one physician's treatment opinions against another's or by threatening to get the requested drug from a "smarter" or "more caring" physician. Treatment recommendations that involve behavioral change, cognitive behavioral therapy, Twelve Step recovery programs, or other nonpharmacological interventions are resisted. The patient may offer financial bribes or sex, or may make outright threats of harm to the physician or his or her property (Longo et al. 2000).

Doctor shopping is a term that describes a patient practice of using at least two and often multiple physicians in an effort to obtain an adequate or an increasing supply of prescriptions for controlled substances. Doctor shoppers often "role-play" with a number of different well-intentioned but possibly naive physicians to obtain multiple prescriptions, which are used personally or sold to support other drug habits (Longo et al. 2000).

Doctor shopping is one of the most common methods of obtaining prescription drugs for legal and illegal use, and many physicians perceive doctor shopping as the major avenue of diversion (Manchikanti 2006). Doctor shopping is most common in emergency department settings, where staff are less likely to know the patient. Frequently, drug-addicted patients seek medical care after-hours and claim to be from out of town (Longo et al. 2000).

The practice of doctor shopping can also involve individuals with legitimate medical needs, such as cancer patients or patients recovering from orthopedic trauma, who travel to several different cities to be seen by various physicians to get prescription medications. Patients practicing doctor shopping may target physicians who are known to readily dispense prescriptions without thorough examinations or screening. Reports exist of individuals collecting thousands of pills during a one-year period and

selling them on the street (Kraman 2004), and of the elderly supplement-
ing their Social Security checks by selling portions of their prescriptions
(Alford 2005).

Doctor shopping has historically been difficult to recognize, but the
increasingly widespread use of computerized prescription monitoring programs by pharmacy networks and managed care companies is making this
type of drug-seeking behavior increasingly difficult (Longo et al. 2000).

Patient Manipulation or Pressure

Although many "conning" tactics seem obvious when described, they can
be used convincingly, especially in the setting of a busy medical office or
emergency department (Wilford 1990).

The Transient Patient

The *transient patient* is from out of town and has lost or has had his or
her medication stolen. The patient attempts to create a sense of urgency
and pressures the physician for an immediate response by claiming intense
pain. Clinical intuition will often alert the physician of the discrepancy
between the levels of observed pain and the self-report of pain. Some
patients' manipulativeness can be detected by observation. For example,
when a physician has the impression that his or her responses are being
studied by the patient as intensely as the physician is studying the
patient's situation, the physician should suspect that the patient is a doctor
shopper or a conning patient. The ordinary patient does not scan the
physician for responses in the same way in which those trying to "con"
may (Wilford 1990).

The Spellbinding Patient

Patients with *pseudologia fantastica* or Munchausen syndrome, or those
who are skilled at deception, can be unusually persuasive compared to
ordinary clinical encounters. When the physician has the feeling that the
patient has extraordinary persuasive and dramatic powers, suspicion that
a manipulator may be present is justified (Wilford 1990).

Likewise, the patient with no interest in diagnosis or follow-up for
further testing and evaluation, or who refuses to see another physician
for consultation, should be suspected. Most manipulative patients shun

real workups and resist attempts to verify history, whereas genuine patients rarely refuse such efforts (Wilford 1990).

Pressure or manipulation is sometimes used to obtain additional medications, more potent or higher dosage formulations, or brand-name drugs because of their higher street value. Patients rarely self-medicate with prescribed drugs that do not produce a high or reward, and they are often quite skilled at projecting their misery and helplessness onto prospective prescribers. A patient who receive an initial "no" (refusal to prescribe by the physician) that is eventually changed to a "yes" (willingness to prescribe) in the face of pressure is considered by some experts to exhibit a classic indicator of prescription drug abuse. Once manipulation or pressure has worked in a given practice, the behavior will likely resurface periodically in that office practice until the physician stops reinforcing the behavior. To deal with patient pressure and manipulation, physicians need to learn to recognize common manipulations and refuse to give in to them (Longo et al. 2000; Parran 1997).

An anecdote involving a drug-seeking patient is provided by the *New York Times.* In an interview with a reporter from the *Times,* an OxyContin addict explained, "It's a slow process, breaking a doctor in. You've got to know how to work him. I'd say: 'I can't take the Vicodins and the Percocets because they're hurting my stomach. Do they have anything that's time released?' The doctor goes, 'Oh, you know what, they've got this new stuff called OxyContin.' And I'd say: 'Oh, yeah? Wow, how's that work?'" Some local doctors, the patient said, knew exactly what was going on, but they needed the business. One started handing out month-long OxyContin prescriptions every two weeks (Tough 2001).

Criminal Activity

In July 2008, the average illicit street price *per milligram* of some of the most sought-after diverted prescription opiates were the following (NDIC 2009):

- hydrocodone (Vicodin, Lortab): $1.90
- methadone: $1.45
- oxycodone (OxyContin, Percocet, Roxicodone): $1.15

Other street values from 2006 are shown in table 4.1.

The high street value of prescription painkillers drives criminal behavior by enticing sellers with highly lucrative profits, and by compelling users to come up with the money needed for their drug of choice.

Prescription drug theft can occur at any point from the manufacturer to the patient. The high demand for prescription drugs is driven by dramatic increases in abuse, and the correspondingly high street prices, as illustrated above, have been fueling a substantial increase in drug theft. Prescription forgery is another common criminal behavior, and is done either by altering the prescription or stealing blank prescription pads in order to write fake prescriptions. Prescription forgery may also occur by calling in prescriptions under a false identity. Legitimate prescriptions are typically altered to increase the quantity of the controlled substance. Pharmacists may participate in prescription drug diversion by selling the controlled substance and then using their database of physicians and patients to write and forge prescriptions to cover their illegal sales. However, most prescription forgery is committed by non-health-care

Table 4.1

Street Values of Diverted Prescription Drugs, 2006

Generic name	Brand name	Brand cost per 100	Street value per 100
Acetaminophen w/Codeine 30 mg	Tylenol #3	$56.49	$800.00
Diazepam 10 mg	Valium 10 mg	$298.04	$1,000.00
Hydromorphone	Dilaudid 4 mg	$88.94	$10,000.00
Methylphenidate	Ritalin	$88.24	$1,500.00
Oxycodone	OxyContin 80 mg	$1,081.36	$8,000.00

(KASPER 2006)

professionals (Wang and Christo 2009; Manchikanti 2006). Prescription forgery is very easy with a word processor and a good printer.

The Diversion of Methadone

Methadone has a long, successful history as a potent painkiller and is a highly effective medication for reducing the morbidity and mortality associated with heroin and other opioid addiction. In the past decade, methadone has emerged as a preferred drug to manage chronic noncancer pain, both as a first-line medication and as a replacement opioid for use in cases where other opioid painkillers have been ineffective. However, recent reports of methadone-related deaths have stirred public concern. Diversion, abuse, and deaths associated with many opioid medications, including methadone, have been prominently featured in the media, and methadone has been described as a dangerous and widely abused "killer drug" (Manchikanti 2006).

In 2001, SAMHSA assumed responsibility from the FDA for the regulation and oversight of the nation's opioid treatment programs, referred to as methadone maintenance clinics. Retail sales of methadone, as measured in grams, increased 812% from 1997 to 2004, an increase second only to oxycodone, with the liquid formulation of methadone seeing the largest increase. In 2002, 68% of methadone purchases were for methadone clinics, with pharmacies purchasing 29%; and within methadone clinics in 2002, 65% of methadone was distributed as liquid, 26% as diskettes, and less than 1% as tablets (CSAT 2004a). Although most methadone is used by methadone clinics, the greatest growth in methadone distribution in recent years—and with it diversion and mortality—originates from its use as a prescription painkiller and its distribution through pharmacies (Manchikanti 2006).

The distribution of methadone to pharmacies, hospitals, and practitioners for legitimate use in pain control increased from 2001 through 2006, with many practitioners beginning to dispense methadone as a pain reliever following the negative publicity surrounding OxyContin's high potential for addiction and abuse (NDIC 2007).

Methadone is diverted in a variety of ways. Wholesale-level quantities of methadone are stolen from delivery trucks and reverse distributors, and midlevel quantities are stolen from businesses such as hospitals and pharmacies. Retail-level quantities are often obtained through traditional prescription drug diversion methods, such as doctor shopping and prescription fraud. Patients being legitimately treated for chronic or cancer pain with methadone represent another source of diversion (NDIC 2007).

Sharing by Family and Friends

One of the most common methods by which controlled substance prescriptions are diverted is through friends and family, often by a person with a legitimate need for a controlled substance who uses only a portion of the prescribed amount and shares the remainder with friends and family. Alternatively, substance abusers, or even curious teenagers, living in the home of someone with a controlled substance prescription may help themselves to the unused portion (Rannazzisi 2006; Manchikanti 2006).

A Naturalistic Study of an Urban Prescription Opioid Diversion Network

Inciardi and colleagues (2009) conducted a groundbreaking qualitative study of the underground economy and the key players involved in diverting, distributing, and using prescription opiates in an urban setting, in this case, Wilmington, Delaware. The author and his colleagues worked on gaining the trust of several key players and gathered information through focus groups and interviews. Among the participants were prescription drug abusers, police, regulatory officials, prescription drug dealers, and pill brokers.

According to the focus group participants, dealers are usually drug abusers who obtain prescription opioids and other drugs through any means necessary to support their own drug habits. Pill brokers, in contrast to the drug dealer, tend to be more organized and do not abuse prescription opioids. Pill brokers often specialize in only one or two drugs, while others buy and sell any type of prescription medication. Pill-brokering operations were described as highly organized and sophisticated enterprises involving a network of patients that divert legitimately acquired medications and often include a given set of doctor shoppers, pain patients, pharmacists, or even physicians.

The prescription opioid most often diverted and abused was hydrocodone, with the biggest diverters being doctor shoppers and students bringing drugs in from out of state. Other players significantly contributing to oxycodone diversion include the elderly and pain patients, pill brokers and dealers, open-air drug markets, family and friends, "script docs" (physicians who knowingly violate the law by writing prescriptions for opioids and other drugs for a fee and without a physical exam), and nurses. Although a few focus group participants had some form of medical insurance, almost all drug purchases from pharmacies, script doctors, and dealers were made with cash.

The focus group members provided details of the different players, what their roles were in the diversion operation, and their typical activities.

The Elderly

Focus group participants consistently stated that many members of the elderly population in Wilmington deceived their physicians with complaints of pain (whether they were in pain or not) to obtain the prescriptions they wanted. Some of these elderly individuals were reportedly abusing the drugs, while most were diverting their medications for economic reasons. Some sold their prescriptions on their own, while others would work with a dealer or pill broker. Generally, the elderly were not drug dealers, but filled their prescriptions and sold part or all of them to a few abusers whom they personally knew, to dealers, or to pill brokers for much below the street value of the drugs. For example, one female prescription drug abuser in her early thirties explained:

> In my neighborhood we have a lot of . . . old people . . . who get these pills prescribed; they get methadone prescribed; they get needles and all that, and that's how they make their money. I have 20 different old people that I can go to [for prescription opioids].

Similarly, a young male polydrug abuser echoed:

> [The elderly] have a lot of 80 milligram Oxys [extended-release oxycodone]; everybody got the big green pills, and everybody had Xanax.

There were old people that were, especially this lady, that was doing like 5 or 6 doctors . . . and getting all kinds of prescription pills. They were just giving them to her. She was just selling them.

And yet another explained:

I've seen a lot of . . . older people who don't have a lot of money get addicted to getting the money from the pills that they sell . . . and they'll go from doctor to doctor, shopping for pills to sell to people.

Pain Patients

The focus group participants were in agreement that many patients who were suffering from serious pain would use part of their prescriptions and sell the rest because they needed cash. Some were dependent on street drugs and would sell or exchange prescription drugs for heroin or crack. Several patients would request additional prescriptions from their pain management specialists, which they would fill and sell to an addict, a drug dealer, or a pill broker. Also common in this group was the selling of unused medications. One male dealer in his early twenties explained:

The people that I knew had [fentanyl patches and fentanyl lollipops]. They received them for back pain, or they were in an accident, and a lot of them were addicts but they wouldn't take their patches and stuff. They would trade the patches for other drugs such as crack.

Also:

I was buying my fentanyl patches from somebody who was getting them prescribed because of back problems. And sometimes they want their crack money so they're going to get rid of their pain pills.

Dealers, Brokers, and Drug Markets

The focus groups consistently reported that pill brokers develop name, address, and medication lists of people they know are willing to sell their prescribed opioids, along with a list of elderly individuals willing to deceive their physicians, have their prescriptions filled by certain local pharmacists, and then sell their pills back to the pill brokers for a fraction of their street value. The pill broker participants confirmed the sophistication of their brokering operations that include strategies such as tracking when their contacts' various prescriptions run out, maintaining a network for contacting these individuals, and arranging for doctor's visits, refills, and transportation as needed. As one prescription drug abuser in his early twenties explained, "Once people [pill brokers] know you take them [prescription opioids], they'll start calling you. 'Oh, it's this time of the month.' Then they . . . wait for that person to get their script. They know exactly in their head what day the script's getting ready to come so they got the patterns down."

Pill brokers and dealers stated that they gathered in open-air drug markets, usually strip mall and pharmacy parking lots, and outside methadone clinics to buy, sell, and trade prescription drugs. A variety of transactions occurred in these markets, including the purchase of prescription drugs for cash, and trades for crack and heroin. Pill brokers also reported buying used fentanyl patches from nurses who have stolen them from pain patients or from disposal containers in hospitals. Some individuals frequenting the drug markets also barter their oxycodone for other opioids or benzodiazepines, typically alprazolam.

Doctor Shopping

Focus group participants indicated that doctor shopping was relatively easy, even in a small state like Delaware; that the vast majority of abusers obtained medications through doctor shopping; and that most reported visiting at least four physicians to obtain sufficient amounts of their desired medications. Clinics and hospital emergency rooms were also reported as locations for doctor shopping.

The most common scenario reported by abusers was to present with a pain complaint, especially back pain because it was fairly easy to simulate.

There was general agreement that most physicians were easy to deceive and manipulate. A male polydrug abuser explained: "I actually rode up here [to Wilmington] with [this lady] one night, and she was getting a lot of bottles of pills. This woman was going to five or six doctors and was manipulating them—pain management doctors and psychologists. How in the world does a 130-pound woman that's in her sixties need ninety Xanax 'bars' [2-mg oblong pills] for a month? She got a bottle full of bars that day." A heavy prescription drug abuser commented: "Along with that accident that I was just telling you about, then came the whole painkiller thing. Like he [another focus group member] was saying about the doctors, it's out of control. I had eight doctors that would give me four or five different kinds of painkillers at one time." Many focus group participants stated that elderly physicians were the most common targets for doctor shopping.

"Script" Docs and Nurses

A few focus group participants reported visits to local "script" docs, although this approach was not widespread. A few had purchased opioids from nurses who stole the drugs from the hospitals and physician offices where they worked, but this too was uncommon among participants.

Other Sources of Prescription Medications

Less common sources of prescription drugs, as indicated by the participants, were friends and family members. However, many participants stated that "medications are everywhere," that "lots of people have leftover meds that they don't need," and that "there is a lot of stealing from medicine cabinets." Others spoke of small shipments of opioids from out of state. The Internet was not reported by any of the participants as a source for prescription opiates.

Sources of Procurement by Teens and College Students

Data from the National Survey on Drug Use and Health (NSDUH) indicate that 56% of people age 12 and older obtain prescription painkillers for nonmedical use from a friend or relative for free, and that 81% of these nonmedical users say that the drugs were prescribed by one doctor. Other NSDUH data regarding the sources of prescription opiates indicated that

18.1% acquired the drugs directly from one doctor, 8.9% bought the drugs from a friend or family member, 5.2% stole them from a friend or family member, 4.1% purchased the drugs from a dealer or stranger, and only 0.5% reported purchasing the prescription opioids on the Internet (NDIC 2009).

Young adults, age 18 to 25, procured prescription painkillers for nonmedical use from the following sources: 53% from a friend or relative for free, 13% from one doctor, and 11% from a friend or relative. Young adult females were more likely than their male counterparts to obtain prescription opiates free from a friend or relative, while males were substantially more likely to purchase the drugs from a friend, relative, dealer, or stranger. Among young adults who met the diagnostic criteria for prescription opiate abuse or dependence, 37% reported their most recent prescription opiates were free from a friend or relative, 20% were purchased from a friend or relative, and 14% were prescribed by a single doctor. The pattern of gender differences in the source of drugs among those meeting criteria for abuse or dependence was similar to that of the larger sample. Interestingly, fewer than 1% of those surveyed obtained their most recent prescription opioid from prescription forgery, Internet purchase, or theft from a health facility (table 4.2) (SAMHSA 2006c).

McCabe and colleagues (2005) administered an Internet survey to 9,161 undergraduate students on the sources of illicitly used prescription drugs. They found that *peer* sources were the most common avenue of supply and, surprisingly, that few respondents reported the Internet as their source of prescription drugs. The authors concluded that the lack of Internet use is explained by the ease in finding abusable prescription medications through other means (McCabe et al. 2005).

Demand Factors Contributing to Increased Prescription Opioid Abuse

The Concept of Opioid Attractiveness

The concept of opioid attractiveness may influence the extent to which a drug is abused. Characteristics that make some drugs more appealing than others include the time to onset following ingestion and the method of

Table 4.2

Method of Obtaining Prescription Opioid for Most Recent Nonmedical Use in Past Year among 18- to 25-Year-Olds

All survey respondents*		Respondents meeting abuse or dependence criteria**	
From a Friend or Relative for Free	53.0%	From a Friend or Relative for Free	37.5%
Prescriptions from One Doctor	12.7%	Bought from a Friend or Relative	19.9%
Bought from a Friend or Relative	10.6%	Prescriptions from One Doctor	13.6%
Bought from a Drug Dealer or Other Stranger	4.8%	Bought from a Drug Dealer or Other Stranger	12.5%
Took from a Friend or Relative without Asking	3.8%	Took from a Friend or Relative without Asking	6.3%
Got Them Some Other Way	2.9%	Prescriptions from More Than One Doctor	2.8%
Prescriptions from More Than One Doctor	1.3%	Got Them Some Other Way	2.3%
Other Unknown or Invalid Source	10.0%	Bought on the Internet	1.3%
		Other Unknown or Invalid Source	1.9%

* The following response options were reported at less than 1% and, therefore, are not shown: "Wrote a Fake Prescription," "Bought on the Internet," and "Stole Them from a Health Facility."

** The following response options were reported at less than 1% and are not shown: "Wrote a Fake Prescription" and "Stole Them from a Health Facility."

(SAMHSA 2006c)

administration (Budman, Serrano, and Butler 2009). Brand-name prescription drugs are routinely worth more on the street than their generic equivalents, because the brand-name drugs are readily recognizable as the "real thing." Generic pills do not enjoy this same status or "purchase power" (Longo et al. 2000). For example, the generic versions of oxycodone ER (extended release) and the fentanyl transdermal patch are diverted less often than the original branded drugs OxyContin and Duragesic (Inciardi et al. 2009).

Attitudinal Factors among Users

The popularity of prescription drugs in the illicit street market is based on abusers' perceptions of these drugs as (1) less stigmatizing, (2) more controlled and therefore less dangerous, and (3) less subject to legal consequences than illegal drugs (Inciardi et al. 2009).

In the Inciardi and colleagues (2009) study, which included a focus group of players involved in drug diversion, the participants agreed that prescription drugs are popular on the street because they are considered more acceptable, less dangerous, and less subject to legal consequences than are illicit drugs. Most also felt that it was easier to rationalize the abuse of prescription medications. For example, in terms of safety, a 23-year-old male emphasized: "I always liked that prescription stuff more because I know what I'm getting; I know the quality, it's predetermined. I know what's in it. I don't have to worry about what I'm snorting or shooting or any of that."

A female abuser in her early twenties also commented on acceptability and lower stigma: "When you're on the street, the person that's doing heroin is a 'junkie.' If you look at a person that's doing Percocets, they would just say, 'Well, I just do Percocets.' You know what I mean? For a long time when I did Percocets and didn't do dope, I looked at people as if they were junkies, but I wasn't."

Another participant reiterated: "I thought it was a safer drug because it was legal. So who cares if I'm abusing it, it's legal, so what are they going to do?" (Inciardi et al. 2009).

Regarding drug desirability, most of the participants said that the fentanyl transdermal patch was the most sought-after prescription opioid. In addition to the potency, this popularity was due to the number of different ways that it could be used, with medication extracted from the patch being injected or snorted as the most common approaches. However, the fentanyl patch was generally less available than other prescription drugs. Also highly sought after, but infrequently obtained, were hydromorphone tablets (Inciardi et al. 2009).

The next most sought-after drug was the OxyContin brand extended-release oxycodone, with prices ranging from $0.40 to $1 per mg, depending on whether the drug was branded or generic. By contrast, the most common and readily available opioid was immediate release (IR) oxycodone, selling for $5 to $10 per pill for both the branded and generic forms. The least expensive and most available prescription drugs on the street were benzodiazepines such as alprazolam and clonazepam—ranging in price from $1 to $3 per pill. The focus group participants expressed little interest in hydrocodone, preferring more potent prescription opioids (Inciardi et al. 2009).

Several focus group participants said that ER oxycodone was becoming more difficult to obtain from some doctors due to recent media attention on the abuse of OxyContin and that other opioids, particularly the fentanyl transdermal patch, were being used in its place (Inciardi et al. 2009).

Among Adolescents

The abuse of prescription medications, referred to as *pharming,* has become normalized in teen culture (Manchikanti 2006). Many teens erroneously believe that abusing prescription or over-the-counter medicines is not harmful, and teens say there is easy access to these drugs through a medicine cabinet at home or at a friend's house or via the Internet. A study by the Partnership Attitude Tracking Study (Pasierb 2006) on teen perception of risk found that

- 40%, or 9.4 million teens surveyed, believed that prescription drugs, even if not prescribed by a doctor, are "much safer" to use than illegal drugs
- 31%, or 7.3 million teens, believed that there is "nothing wrong" with using prescription drugs without a prescription "once in a while"

- 29%, or 6.8 million teens, believed prescription painkillers, even if not prescribed by a doctor, are not addictive
- more than half of teens (55%, or 13 million) do not strongly agree that using cough medicine to get high is risky (Pasierb 2006; Manchikanti 2006)

Parental Unawareness

Although today's parents are the most drug-experienced in history, they often do not understand the drug abuse behavior among today's teens. In part, this may be because they are looking for the traditional signs of illegal drug use and are consequentially failing to detect the signs of modern-day prescription drug abuse (Pasierb 2006). This disconnect between parents and teens on pharming has been documented: Only 1% of parents said it is "extremely or very likely" that their own teen has tried a prescription painkiller, but 21% of teens admitted trying this type of drug to get high (Pasierb 2006). The same holds true for prescription stimulants: 2% of parents said it is "extremely or very likely" that their own teen has used them to get high, whereas 10% of teens actually have (Pasierb 2006; Manchikanti 2006).

Children who learn about the risk of drugs from their parents are much less likely to use drugs than teens whose parents don't discuss this issue. And although most parents of teens claim they have talked to their child about the dangers of drugs, fewer than one-third of teens (31% or 7.4 million) state they "learn a lot about the risks of drugs" from their parents. Research shows that parents are also the first place that teens turn for information about the risk of drugs (Pasierb 2006). Fifty-six percent of teens reported that they talk to their mothers and 45% would turn to their fathers when they have a question about drugs (Manchikanti 2006; Pasierb 2006).

Advertising and Advocacy

Several aspects of marketing and advertising contribute to the demand for controlled substances and prescription opioids. These include increased direct-to-consumer advertising, which fosters the view that prescription drugs are integral to consumers' lives; aggressive marketing techniques with pharmaceutical companies providing gifts and information to physicians;

and patient advocacy groups that demand opioids for nonmalignant pain and advance the position that pain should be aggressively treated in all cases (Manchikanti 2006).

SUMMARY

It is extremely easy to obtain prescription opioids and our youth do not recognize the risks associated with their recreational use. The availability of these medications has contributed to the current problem—prescription medications are the fourth most common drug of abuse, behind nicotine, alcohol, and marijuana. The tremendous potential profits from selling prescription opioids ensure a long-standing problem, especially since otherwise law-abiding citizens are contributing to the illicit drug market to make ends meet. The ease of access to these drugs is directly related to the dramatic increase in opioid prescriptions and has resulted in an increase in abuse, dependence, associated medical problems, and death.

Characteristics of Abuse and Dependence

Emergence of the Modern Theory of Opioid Addiction

Two researchers, Vincent Dole and Marie Nyswander, theorized that methadone could block craving for opioids and subsequently stabilize the lives of people addicted to heroin and other opioid drugs. Perhaps their greatest achievement was to shift the paradigm of addictive behavior from a moralistic weakness of character and psychological failing to that of a chronic *metabolic disease* (Dole and Nyswander 1967; Joseph and Woods 2006).

Dr. Nyswander wrote several papers about her experiences treating addicts, as well as the book *The Drug Addict as a Patient* in 1956. At the time, considering addicts as patients was a revolutionary concept in the United States, since heroin addicts were relegated to the prison system or prison-like hospitals (Joseph and Woods 2006). Dole and Nyswander's *metabolic theory* evolved from a seminal paper published in 1967, *Heroin Addiction: A Metabolic Disease.* In this paper, they introduced factors supporting their argument, such as neurological susceptibility, an altered biological response to opioid drugs that results in continued use, a protracted abstinence syndrome, and a craving that precipitated relapse. According to Dole, the specific hunger for opioid drugs that led to relapse was a symptom of a metabolic alteration within the central nervous system and was unrelated to the addict's psychological profile, social class, or emotional state (Dole and Nyswander 1967; Joseph and Woods 2006).

In 1970, Dole published the article "The Biochemistry of Addiction," in which he predicted the existence of opioid receptors in the brain, their location and density, and the technology needed to isolate them. This endogenous opioid receptor system was discovered within a few years of his prediction, and Dole stated in this paper that the metabolic changes responsible for the opioid craving now appeared to be associated with impairment or deficit in the function of this yet-to-be discovered opioid receptor system (Dole 1988; Joseph and Woods 2006). In 1994, Dole summarized the metabolic theory of addiction that had evolved over the past forty years (Joseph and Woods 2006):

> Craving for opiate drugs is a symptom of a deficiency in function of the
>
> natural opiate-like substances in the brain. To be sure, sociological and
>
> psychological forces enter into the making of an addict, but these factors
>
> determine exposure—whether or not addictive drugs are available in the
>
> environment and whether a person chooses to experiment with them. In
>
> any person with repeated exposure to a narcotic drug, the brain adapts
>
> and becomes pharmacologically dependent on a continuing input. In
>
> some susceptible persons—fortunately a minority of the population—
>
> the adaptation becomes fixed and with repeated use a regular input of
>
> narcotic becomes a necessity. The experimenter has become an addict.
>
> (Dole 1994)

According to Dole's theory of addiction, then, social, psychological, and biological elements are combined, with each playing a defined and interrelated role. Psychological and social elements may be responsible for experimental and initial use, but eventually biological forces take over, regardless of the psychosocial elements responsible for experimentation or initial use. Continued craving, relapse to opioid use after a period of

abstinence, and tolerance associated with addiction have biological components and operate independently of willpower and a person's psychological
makeup. This theory has two important implications: The basic characteristics of a continued addiction are biologically influenced; and in most
cases, the resolution of the psychological or social problems that motivated
the person to initially use substances does not subsequently resolve drug
cravings or other biological components of an addiction (Magura and
Rosenblum 2000; Joseph and Woods 2006).

Natural History of Opioid Addiction

Most people who become addicted to prescription opioids do not experience a full-blown addiction right away. Rather, progressive changes in the
patterns of drug use occur over time as the addiction progresses from
experimentation to regular use, to compulsive use, and then to drug use
just to feel normal. This progression is referred to as the *natural history* of
opioid addiction. In fact, contrary to popular belief, only about 23% of
those who use heroin become addicted to it (NIDA 2010).

Research has repeatedly found that once people vulnerable to addiction
begin using opioids, drug use often escalates to more severe levels, with
repeated cycles of stopping and starting use over extended periods—the
same as addiction to other substances. This process has been referred to as
a *drug use career, dependence career,* or *addiction career* (Frykholm 1985;
Hser, Anglin, and Powers 1993; Maddux and Desmond 1981; McGlothlin,
Anglin, and Wilson 1977; Simpson and Sells 1982; Stephens 1991) while
cycles of treatment, abstinence, and relapse have been called the treatment
career (Hser et al. unpublished; Senay 1984).

Although drug use careers may vary widely in terms of length, pattern,
ultimate outcome (Anglin 1998), and time from initiation of drug use to
daily use to serious physical and psychological addiction (Schwartz 1998),
the opioid abuser tends to move through four stages of addiction in a predictable manner: initiation, maintenance or continuation, detoxification
and withdrawal, and relapse (van den Brink and Haasen 2006). Each stage
involves specific brain chemicals (neurotransmitters) and brain structures
and activation of specific brain circuits. Understanding these different

processes helps us develop intervention and treatment approaches that are more targeted and specific to the stage of addiction (van den Brink and Haasen 2006).

Initiation

Many factors—genetic, individual, and environmental—help determine whether a person who experiments with opioid drugs will continue taking them long enough to become dependent or addicted. The opioids' ability to provide intense feelings of pleasure is a critical reason why some people continue to use them after experimentation. When opioid molecules travel through the bloodstream into the brain, they attach to specialized proteins, called opioid receptors, on the surface of certain brain cells (neurons). The binding of these molecules with their target receptors triggers the same brain chemical response in the brain's reward center that occurs with anything that causes intense pleasure or is intended to be reinforcing to survival itself. This is the part of the brain that ensures our survival—by reinforcing acts like eating, drinking fluids, caring for our babies, and having sex (for survival of the species). All rewarding and survival-based activities result in release of dopamine in the mesolimbic system of the brain. Dopamine signals the importance of the activity and results in repetition of those acts that cause its release, reinforcing survival-related behaviors and keeping us and our species alive. All drugs of abuse trigger the release of dopamine in amounts exceeding those released by normal activities that provide pleasure or keep us alive. Just like other drugs of abuse, opioids cause excess dopamine release in the reward center, also called the mesolimbic system of our brains, signaling the brain at a subconscious level in those prone to addiction that something extremely important has taken place and it needs to be repeated. Although opioids are prescribed to relieve pain, when they activate these reward processes they can create a powerful motivation for repeated use simply for pleasure (Kosten and George 2002).

The way different classes of drugs make us feel differs dramatically. People who use cocaine do not experience the same type of intoxication as those who use opioids; the drugs alter different parts of the brain and interact with different cells and receptors to cause a particular type of intoxication. However, in the end, both classes of drugs—in fact all addicting drugs—cause release of excess dopamine in the mesolimbic system, contributing to the risk of addiction.

Scientists have determined how opioids cause the release of excess dopamine. Opioid molecules bind to the mu-opioid receptors found on the surface of gamma-aminobutyric acid (GABA) cells in the ventral tegmental area (VTA) and the nucleus accumbens (NAcc). When the mu-opioid receptor is stimulated by occupancy of an opioid molecule, it sends a signal that blocks the actions of the GABA neurons that normally inhibit the activity of dopamine neurons in the VTA. When the GABA cells activity is blocked or made inactive, a surge of excess dopamine occurs in the NAcc and other adjacent brain structures (van den Brink and van Ree 2003). As a result of this cascade of brain chemicals, the user experiences rewarding effects (Xi and Stein 2002).

Again, this activation of chemical pathways by the opioid drug occurs within the mesolimbic reward system, of which the VTA and NAcc are part. It also activates other areas of the mesolimbic system, creating a lasting record, or memory, that links these intense feelings of pleasure with the circumstances and environment in which they occurred. These memories are called *conditioned associations* and often lead to intense drug cravings when the opioid user is around people, places, or things associated with getting high. These cravings may be so powerful that, even when the opioid abuser has resolved to stop using, they overwhelm the person's ability to remain abstinent (Kosten and George 2002).

During the initiation phase of addiction, *reinforcement* occurs—the overwhelmingly pleasurable drug effect that compels the user to recapture the experience. This reinforcement process during the initiation phase is mediated by mu-opioid receptors and dopamine in the VTA and NAcc and other parts of the mesolimbic system which result in conditioned responses and drug craving (van den Brink and Haasen 2006). Everyone exposed to opioids experiences excess dopamine release in the mesolimbic system of the brain. However, most people do not become addicted to opioids after such exposure. Although experts are not yet entirely sure why this is so, it may be related to altered function of dopamine receptors in those predisposed to addiction, either secondary to genetic alteration or changed by life experience or the drugs themselves, which ultimately triggers addiction. To neurobiologists interested in addiction, this is the Holy Grail: explaining how some people become addicted when exposed to these drugs, while most do not.

Maintenance or Continuation

During the early stages of addiction, stimulation of the brain's reward system is the primary reason that some people take the drugs repeatedly. However, this repetitive drive, or compulsion, to use opioids eventually grows beyond a simple drive for pleasure. This increased compulsion is also related to the development of tolerance and dependence (Kosten and George 2002).

Prolonged use of increasingly higher doses of opioid drugs changes the brain so that it functions more or less normally when the drug is present and abnormally when the drug is removed. This alteration in the brain results in both opioid tolerance (the need to take higher and higher doses to achieve the same drug effect) and opioid dependence (susceptibility to withdrawal symptoms when use of the drug is suddenly decreased or abruptly stopped). Withdrawal symptoms occur only in users who have developed tolerance (Kosten and George 2002).

Let's briefly consider the difference between physical dependence to opioids and addiction to opioids. Physical dependence will occur in anyone who is prescribed opioid painkillers for pain control over an extended period of time; it is the result of the brain and body adjusting to the constant presence of opioids. Addiction only occurs in a minority of individuals who regularly use opioid medications. These users experience an overwhelming initial high—euphoria, relaxation, well-being, and "bliss"—followed by a craving to recapture this effect, compulsive use of the drug, and continued use despite harmful consequences.

When tolerance to opioids develops, the drug becomes less effective in producing the desired effects. Euphoria is the effect that most opioid users seek, but it's also the effect most likely to diminish with regular use (White and Irvine 1999). The brain process that underlies the development of tolerance is thought to be the desensitization of opioid receptors (Gutstein and Akil 2006). The receptors have been repeatedly overstimulated, resulting in a cellular response, most likely the result of altered or removed receptor sites, in an attempt to limit the overstimulation. The cells are trying to protect themselves from the overstimulation.

Opioid tolerance occurs, then, because the brain cells with opioid receptors gradually become less responsive to the activation that normally occurs when an opioid molecule binds to the opioid receptor on the cell. If there are fewer opioid receptors, or their function has been altered, the cells will not have the same degree of stimulation; the response will be dampened. Chronic opioid users need higher doses of opioids to stimulate the VTA brain cells in the mesolimbic reward system into releasing a larger amount of dopamine into the NAcc (Tso and Wong 2003). In other words, more drug is needed to produce the desired drug effect compared with earlier periods of drug use (Kosten and George 2002). These changes in the sensitivity of the opioid receptor to the chronic presence of opioid molecules bathing brain cells on a daily basis occur at the molecular and cellular level, and have far-reaching consequences when the user attempts to stop taking opioids and remain drug free (Tso and Wong 2003). Tolerance also affects how the drug is taken. As tolerance develops, the dose and/or route of administration often change as the user tries to achieve the sensation of the high, with progression to IV use a frequent outcome (Schwartz 1998).

As we have seen, in early addiction the intense pleasure that occurs when the brain's reward system is activated by opioids can promote continued drug use. Frequent and prolonged use of the drug leads to opioid dependence. When dependence develops, the opioid user begins using the drug more often to avoid unpleasant withdrawal symptoms. With prolonged use, additional long-lasting changes occur in the brain that may underlie the compulsive drug-seeking behavior and the negative consequences that are the hallmarks of addiction (Kosten and George 2002). During maintenance use of an opioid, the brain functions closer to normal in the presence of the drug, but is remarkably abnormal without it.

Withdrawal and Detoxification

Opioid *withdrawal* refers to the process of discontinuing the opioid, either gradually or suddenly. The opioid *withdrawal syndrome* is a group of extremely unpleasant and distressing symptoms that emerge shortly after discontinuation of opioids. *Detoxification* refers to the medically managed withdrawal from opioids used for a smooth transition to a drug-free state. The opiate withdrawal syndrome is often simply called *opioid withdrawal.*

Opioid withdrawal is one of the most powerful factors driving opioid dependence and addictive behaviors. Treatment of the patient's withdrawal symptoms is based on understanding how withdrawal is related to the brain's adjustment to the long-term presence of opioids (Kosten and George 2002). Opioid withdrawal is not a medically dangerous situation; it does not run the risk of fatalities. However, it is similar to a severe flu and the addict may feel like dying.

Many of the most distressing symptoms of opioid withdrawal stem from changes in another important brain system located at the base of the brain—the locus ceruleus (LC). Normally, cells in the LC produce the chemical norepinephrine and send it to other parts of the brain where it stimulates wakefulness, breathing, blood pressure, and alertness. Using opioid drugs suppresses the activity of these cells in the LC, resulting in drowsiness, slowed breathing rate, and low blood pressure. With long-term opioid use, these cells adjust to the continuous presence and effect of the drug by increasing their activity level, thereby releasing higher amounts of norepinephrine needed for normal function. The person feels fairly normal during long-term opioid use because these LC cells have counteracted the drug effect. However, when opioids are removed from the brain during withdrawal, these cells appear hyperactive because the opioid is no longer in the brain to suppress their activity. Anxiety, muscle cramps, tremors, and diarrhea are all the result of this rebound in LC norepinephrine activity (van den Brink and Haasen 2006; Kosten and George 2002).

Still other areas in the brain also contribute to withdrawal symptoms, including the brain's reward system (discussed earlier). Changes in the reward system that result from chronic opioid use may prevent the individual from obtaining pleasure from normally rewarding nondrug activities (Kosten and George 2002).

Relapse Following Sustained Absence

Professionals who work with people trying to recover from opioid addiction have long realized that these individuals are more vulnerable to stress than most people. In fact, research has found that physical and emotional stress can trigger drug cravings in addicts (e.g., Shaham, Erb, and Stewart 2000). One possible explanation for this is that a sensitivity to stress may contribute to the opioid user's desire to take drugs in the first place, and to the subsequent compulsion to keep taking them (Kosten and George 2002).

Many heroin addicts, when asked what happens when they "kick the habit," describe the classic withdrawal syndrome—nausea, vomiting, aches and pains, yawning, sneezing, and so on. However, when asked about their experiences after physical withdrawal, they describe an equally specific "post-withdrawal syndrome"—a fluctuating, unstable combination of anxiety, depression, and craving for the drug. The craving is not constant, but seems to come and go in waves of varying intensity—for months and even years after being free from opiate use. This craving is particularly likely to return in moments of emotional stress. An intense wave of craving may overpower the addict's ability to remain abstinent; drug-seeking behavior may follow and the person relapses to opioid use. Many addicts, when asked how they feel right after they resumed the opioid, report feeling "normal" again—they find temporary relief from the chronic post-withdrawal symptoms of anxiety, depression, and craving (Brecher 1972).

It is this fact—that an addict takes his or her drug of choice in order to feel "normal"—that is perhaps the most difficult concept of addiction for a nonaddict to understand and believe. Many assume that the addict enjoys the daily use of the drug. Yet, when asked, most opioid addicts cannot recall the last time drug use was enjoyable. It is not the intoxication that drives the addiction; after a certain point daily use becomes a drudgery and its own form of torture. This is consistent with other known behavioral and biological aspects of addiction and indicates that when addicts relapse to their drug of choice early in recovery, they are not necessarily seeking pleasure as much as a return to a "normal" mood and state of mind (Brecher 1972).

Scientists have also identified the regions of the brain that appear to be involved in the process of relapse. They include the orbitofrontal cortex, the anterior cingulate gyrus, and the amygdala. The brain chemicals involved in this process are norepinephrine and corticotropin-releasing hormone. These two brain chemicals help make up the brain stress response system and are involved in one form of relapse, the stress-induced relapse. Other brain chemicals are involved with relapses due to craving triggered from being around reminders of drug use, such as the people, places, and things the person associated with drug using. The neurotransmitters involved in this type of relapse include GABA and glutamate. These two brain chemicals are part of the brain system that is involved in compulsive and habitual behavior (van den Brink and Haasen 2006).

The "Changed Set-Point" Model of Opioid Relapse

According to the *changed set-point* model of opioid addiction, chronic abuse of opioids alters a biological set point, or baseline. Researchers have proposed several versions of the changed set-point model, and all are based on the altered activity of the dopamine cells in the VTA and norepinephrine cells in the LC during the early phases of withdrawal and abstinence from opioids (Kosten and George 2002).

One variant, proposed by George Koob, one of the leading researchers in the neurobiology of addiction, proposes that cells in the brain's mesolimbic reward system are naturally "set" to release enough dopamine in the NAcc to produce a normal level of pleasure. Koob and his colleague (Koob and LeMoal 2001) suggest that opioid use leads to addiction by changing this set point, so that the release of dopamine is reduced when normally pleasurable activities occur and opioids are not present. This change would limit our feelings of pleasure secondary to natural reinforcing activities, and by comparison enhance that of the drug. Another set point is believed to occur in the LC such that release of the brain stress chemical norepinephrine is increased during withdrawal, as described earlier (Kosten and George 2002).

A third variation of the set-point model emphasizes the opioid addict's sensitivity to environmental cues that trigger cravings (Breiter et al. 1997; Robinson and Berridge 2000). During periods when the drug is not available, even when the addict is not in a surrounding associated with drug use, the person still remembers drug use and focuses on it, resulting in desire or craving for the drug that may lead to relapse (Kosten and George 2002).

Prescription Opioids as a "Gateway" to Heroin

Ever since the epidemic in prescription opioid abuse became known to law enforcement, public health, medical, and addiction professionals, there has been great concern over the possibility that abuse, and even casual use of prescription opioids, will lead either to the use of heroin or to a lifetime of substance abuse. Some of this concern has been fueled by stories in the media. For example, a user in rural Appalachia told a reporter from the *New York Times* investigating the epidemic of OxyContin abuse:

> I've always said that I'd never ever touch heroin. But then Oxys came along and that's the same thing, just cleaner. And that got me into shooting dope. If I'd never touched OxyContin, I wouldn't have done heroin.

> (TOUGH 2001)

Returning to the naturalistic study conducted by Inciardi and colleagues (2009), the wealth of information gained from the study participants allowed the researchers to address several questions related to the abuse of diverted prescription opioids. One of these questions relates to the speculation in both the scientific literature and the media that for many abusers, prescription drugs served as a first step or "gateway" to additional substance abuse. Inciardi and colleagues found that all of the focus group participants reported abusing alcohol and marijuana long before they began experimenting with prescription drugs. However, many also said that prescription opioids were a gateway to heroin use. For example, one male heroin user in his early twenties stated: "I started with Percocets and ended up shooting 10 bags of heroin a day." Another 23-year-old male reported: "It led me into heroin. When I was in junior high my grandfather had cancer and he had Percocet and morphine pills, and after he died my grandma still had a lot of his pill bottles around. I . . . started taking them, and . . . after that I was hooked." Others echoed this theme as well: "They [prescription pills] are like just as strong as dope and weed. They are really gateway drugs. They get you there. They get you into that scene."

Several focus group participants also explained that the movement from prescription opioids to heroin was due to the high cost of prescription opioids on the street. For example, a female heroin user in her early thirties explained: "When I first started doing drugs, I started taking the pills, like Xanax, Oxys, Percocets, anything that was prescription. After that I progressed into heroin and cocaine because . . . sometimes the prescription drugs are real expensive. Most pills like an Oxy can be $40. So it was just getting too expensive for me."

A male in his early twenties added: "I never really considered myself an addict, . . . but the OxyContin—that's what led me into an addiction with heroin. After a couple months I thought I was okay with them, but I finally found out I was a junkie."

The study by Inciardi and colleagues indicates that the abuse of prescription opioids such as OxyContin may lead to heroin abuse among individuals who have shown signs of drug abuse or dependence before they began abusing prescription opioids. It is much less likely that a person without previous drug or alcohol abuse will progress to heroin from OxyContin or other prescription opioid abuse. These conclusions by Inciardi and his colleagues have also been reached repeatedly in other studies: The abuse of OxyContin is rarely the initiating factor leading to the abuse of other drugs (Sees et al. 2005); patients diagnosed with OxyContin dependence have high rates of substance abuse that predated the use of OxyContin (Potter et al. 2004); and people without a history of drug or alcohol abuse are unlikely to become addicted to prescription painkillers when they are prescribed for legitimate purposes (Edlund et al. 2007).

Regular opioid use causes tolerance and a yearning for the intense intoxication experienced during initial use. Heroin addicts sometimes refer to this as "chasing the dragon," trying to find the high they once experienced and can no longer attain. Daily use becomes mundane, almost like a job. Advancing to intravenous use of heroin is sometimes an attempt to override tolerance and experience a new intensity of intoxication, similar to the initial use of opioids.

Evidence That Opioid Addiction Is a Medical Disorder

For decades, people addicted to opioids were thought to have a lack of motivation, willpower, or character. Yet careful study of the natural history of opioid addiction and research of addiction at the genetic, molecular, neuronal, and epidemiological levels have proven that opioid addiction is a medical disorder characterized by predictable signs and symptoms. Here are some other arguments for classifying opioid addiction as a medical disorder (NIH 1997):

- Despite different cultural, ethnic, and socioeconomic backgrounds, people who are opioid-addicted show a distinct pattern in the medical history, signs, and symptoms of their use.
- There is a tendency for people addicted to opioids to relapse after periods of abstinence.
- The person addicted to opioids experiences cravings for opioids that can result in repeated relapse even in the presence of powerful social consequences and strong motivation to stop.
- Continuous use of opioids during the course of addiction causes specific changes to key brain regions.

Biological and Behavioral Characteristics of Opioid Abuse and Dependence

The abuse of opioids produces a consistent cluster of effects that are observable to others (signs) and are experienced by the user (symptoms). These include the following:

Signs of opioid intoxication	Symptoms of opiate intoxication
• constricted pupils (dilated in the case of meperidine use)	• euphoria
• drowsiness, "nodding off"	• apathy
• decreased respiration and heart rate	• dysphoria
• pulmonary edema	• psychomotor agitation or retardation
• slurred speech	• impaired social judgment
• impaired attention and memory	• impaired occupational functioning
• stupor and coma	

(Vukmir 2004)

Using opioids intravenously produces intense tranquility, euphoria, analgesia, and clouded awareness of one's surroundings. These effects follow the "rush" that occurs immediately after the IV injection (Schwartz 1998).

Acute and Chronic Effects of Opioid Abuse and Dependence

Infectious Disease

Infectious complications from opioid use generally stem from injecting the drug using contaminated needles, which spreads viruses and bacteria causing blood-borne diseases. An estimated 60% to 90% of IV users have contracted the virus hepatitis C; other common infectious diseases include HIV, hepatitis B, and common bacterial infections such as staphylococcus aureus. Cellulitis and abscesses around the injection site, pneumonia, bacteremia (Schwartz 1998), and bacterial endocarditis are the result of injecting bacteria into the blood. Among people infected with HIV in the

United States, more than one-third have injected opioids and more than 25% reported sharing needles (Havens, Walker, and Leukefeld 2007).

Endocrine/Metabolic Effects

Chronic opioid abuse affects multiple endocrine functions and is associated with hypogonadism, adrenal dysfunction, reduced bone density, and growth-hormone abnormalities (Cooper, Brown, and Dobs 2003).

Cognitive Effects

Cognitive impairment may both contribute to and be a consequence of opioid abuse and dependence in at least two ways: (1) people with certain cognitive defects, such as poor impulse control, are at a greater risk of drug abuse, and (2) cognitive impairment may interfere with the addict's ability to learn and participate in drug treatment programs that have an educational and cognitive emphasis (Rogers and Robbins 2001).

During the acute effect of opioids, users' ability to work safely or drive a car may be impaired. This impairment does not worsen or continue with methadone patients after they have developed a tolerance to the drug over a period of months or years (Specka et al. 2000). However, this assumes methadone patients are using the same dose on a daily basis. If they chose to take twice as much as usual, or add another opioid, they would most likely become intoxicated and could experience impairment.

It is not yet known how long the cognitive effects of opioid use last or what cause them. In one study, where opioid addicts were maintained on methadone long enough to have developed tolerance to the sedating effects of the drug, cognitive functioning more or less equaled that of healthy non-addicts, when education and background were considered. This means that methadone-maintained patients may be as capable as healthy people in job performance, if the minimum background requirements are not extremely high, and if the patient is stable in his or her abstinence from other opioids and other drugs of abuse (Specka et al. 2000). Other studies have suggested that cognitive impairments are linked with methadone use, but could not prove the impairments were caused by methadone. They may have been pre-existing, or secondary to long-term opioid use prior to methadone (Mintzer 2002; Verdejo et al. 2005).

Opioid Overdose

The possible factors that result in an opioid overdose include a lack of tolerance, the interaction between the opioid with other central nervous system (CNS) depressants, or a systemic factor (Warner-Smith et al. 2001). In fatal overdoses, instant death is uncommon, which suggests that intervention is possible in most cases. However, when in the company of someone who has overdosed, other users often do not try to get help, usually because they're afraid of involving the police (Darke and Hall 2003).

The symptoms of an opioid overdose include mental clouding, sedation and then stupor or coma, constricted pupils, an abnormally slow breathing rate, diminished response to painful stimuli, and mottled cooled skin. Respiratory depression—the most feared overdose symptom and almost always the cause of death from an opioid overdose—is the result of the opioid's direct suppression of the brain stem respiratory center. This leads to slowed and shallow breathing, and a greatly reduced volume of air that is inhaled and exhaled (Schwartz 1998). Ultimately, the inadequate oxygen levels cannot sustain life.

The aftermath of a nonfatal opioid overdose can include conditions involving the lungs secondary to the accumulation of fluid in the lung, or pneumonia; cardiac complications such as abnormal heart rhythm, loss of function of the heart muscle, and reduced red blood cell count; breakdown of muscle tissue; and brain damage from lack of oxygen available to the brain (Warner-Smith et al. 2001).

Although partial opioid agonists such as buprenorphine have less effect on respiration, these drugs may still produce potentially fatal respiratory depression if taken with other depressant drugs (White and Irvine 1999), especially high doses of benzodiazepines.

Opioid Withdrawal and Relapse to Opioid Use

A measurable withdrawal syndrome can occur even after a single dose of morphine. Physical dependence to opioids is assessed by observing the emergence of withdrawal following discontinuation of opioids, or through the administration of an opioid antagonist such as naloxone (Noda and Nabeshima 2004), which blocks opioid receptors and thereby prevents the opioid from having an effect.

The signs of opioid withdrawal include the following (Vukmir 2004):

- dilated pupils
- runny nose
- watery eyes
- goose bumps
- nausea
- vomiting
- diarrhea
- yawning
- muscle cramps

The symptoms of opioid withdrawal include the following:

- restlessness
- verbalization of complaints
- elevated vital signs

Although the biology that causes opioid withdrawal is not fully understood, several brain chemical systems are believed to play a large role. These include the dopamine, acetylcholine, norepinephrine, and glutamate systems (Noda and Nabeshima 2004). An area of the brain called the extended amygdala is strongly linked to the negative emotional aspect of withdrawal from chronic exposure to a number of drugs, including opioids (Harris and Gewirtz 2005).

Acute Opioid Withdrawal

Chronic opioid use is associated with physical dependence and a withdrawal syndrome when use of the drug is abruptly stopped. In general, the shorter-acting opioids tend to produce briefer, more intense withdrawal symptoms, while longer-acting opioids produce a withdrawal syndrome that is more drawn out.

Withdrawal symptoms from an opioid such as morphine or oxycodone result when opioid molecules depart from the mu-opioid receptors. Typical symptoms of withdrawal include agitation, anxiety, goose bumps, rapid heart rate, mild hypertension, and pupil dilation. The initial symptoms include yawning, itching, irritability, and insomnia, as well as a runny nose, tearing eyes, sweating, vomiting, and diarrhea.

As symptoms progress, increases in vital signs, pulse, blood pressure, and respiration rate are observed. At the peak of opiate withdrawal, intense anxiety, tremors, shakes, smooth and skeletal muscle cramps, and joint and deep bone pain of varying degrees begin to manifest (Schwartz 1998).

Post-acute (Protracted) Withdrawal and Relapse Vulnerability

Opioid addiction is a chronic relapsing disorder characterized by compulsive drug seeking and compulsive use. The psychological dependence associated with opioid addiction is complex. Long after the physical need for the drug has passed, the addict may continue to think and talk about the use of drugs and feel strange or overwhelmed by daily activities without being under the influence of drugs. There is a high probability of relapse following withdrawal from opioids when neither the physical environment nor the behavioral motivators that contributed to the abuse have been altered.

As described above, important changes in the brain occur during and following both opioid addiction and withdrawal that are believed to heighten this vulnerability to relapse. Animal models of addiction and withdrawal have helped us understand the experience. Aston-Jones and Harris highlight in their review article our current understanding of factors that contribute to relapse, which may be associated with post-acute withdrawal (Aston-Jones and Harris 2004). Abstinence from chronic drug use results in ill-defined feelings of distress, anxiety, or malaise that can only be alleviated by a return to use of an opioid. Continued drug use is rewarding not only because it stimulates the reward circuitry in the brain, but also because it greatly reduces the awful feelings associated with post-acute withdrawal, thereby intensifying the overall positive reinforcement (Aston-Jones and Harris 2004). In other words, the person in post-acute withdrawal is anxious and more susceptible to stress. Return to opioid use relieves the anxiety, which is pleasant, thereby reinforcing, so use becomes more likely. Basically, people relapse in order to feel better.

Chronic opioid abuse also reduces one's ability to experience pleasure and reward from nondrug sources. Unable to enjoy previously pleasurable activities or feeling dysphoric or down serves to increase the person's incentive to use opioids (Aston-Jones and Harris 2004).

Taken together, the heightened risk of relapse during the post-acute withdrawal period may involve two different processes: prolonged and elevated anxiety leading to the desire to resume opioid use to alleviate the unpleasant emotional state, and the chronic difficulty in experiencing normal pleasure or happiness, which can motivate the user to seek the pleasurable effect of the opioid (Aston-Jones and Harris 2004).

Research Findings

As mentioned earlier, the people, places, and things associated with drug using may trigger a desire to use in addicts. This process, called *cue reactivity,* is related to craving but it is not entirely clear just how. However, researchers have been able to identify the processes occurring in the brains of addicts during cue reactivity.

Daglish and colleagues (2001) examined the brain systems that may be involved in craving. They investigated the brain mechanisms of environmental triggers by studying a group of abstinent opioid addicts (average clean time eight months) who were played a tape narrating a craving episode while undergoing a PET scan. These results were compared with PET scans taken while the participants were listening to neutral material. The researchers were able to induce cravings in 67% (eight out of twelve) of the participants, and the PET images revealed consistent patterns: all participants who reported drug craving showed an activation of the left orbitofrontal cortex. Also, the intensity of activity in this brain region corresponded with the intensity of the participant's craving. Previous research has linked the brain's orbitofrontal cortex to the reward system (Koob 1992), which plays an important role in anticipation and reinforcement (Hugdahl et al. 1995; Rolls 1996; Thorpe, Rolls, and Maddison 1983), and suggests that the orbitofrontal cortex may play a role in evaluating the motivational value of stimuli and in labeling the emotional experience of craving (London et al. 2000). Research has also shown that dysfunction in this region of the brain is associated with compulsive behavior and with increased motivation to obtain a drug of abuse (Volkow and Fowler 2000; Daglish et al. 2001). Although craving has yet to be fully defined, these studies provide a framework for our current understanding.

What Is the True Potential of Abuse/Dependence of Legitimately Prescribed Opioid Drugs?

Underuse versus Overuse of Opioid Analgesics

There is broad consensus that patients with acute and chronic pain have often received inadequate pain control, because treating physicians fear creating addiction. This approach of limited pain treatment was demonstrated in a survey, which found that 35% of Canadian family physicians reported they would never prescribe opioids for moderate to severe chronic pain, and 37% identified addiction as a major barrier to prescribing opioids. These results reflect attitudes among physicians that may lead to undertreatment of pain and unnecessary suffering among patients (Kahan et al. 2006). In response to this, the Joint Commission on Accreditation of Healthcare Organizations (JCAHO) and other similar organizations have enacted new accreditation standards stating that pain should be viewed as the fifth vital sign to be assessed whenever other vital signs are measured (Ling, Wesson, and Smith 2005). The subjective experience of pain became the measure used by health care professionals to guide treatment efforts.

However, along with the growing concern about the undertreatment of pain and the underuse of opioids in pain treatment, there is also a renewed concern about prescription opioid addiction and overdose deaths (Ling, Wesson, and Smith 2005), especially in the aftermath of the explosion in OxyContin prescriptions and the abuse and diversion that followed. The disparate concerns regarding undertreatment of pain and facilitation of addiction are underscored by the fact that until recently, pain management and addiction specialists rarely communicated with each other, and each group held a separate point of view. The pain-management physicians rightly concern themselves with alleviation of pain and have traditionally underestimated the rate of addiction among their patients, with such patients often simply dismissed from further care. Addiction specialists, on the other hand, seldom encounter pain patients whose quality of life is vastly improved by opioids, but instead see failed patients from pain-treatment programs (Ling, Wesson, and Smith 2005). Acute pain secondary to injury and surgery responds extremely well to opioids. However, compounding the quandary is the treatment of chronic pain. It is not yet clear whether chronic pain—lasting more than six months—is successfully treated with opioids (Martell et al. 2007). Yet opioids are the most common treatment used.

Corresponding Increases in Abuse with Increased Prescribing of Prescription Opioids

Until the 1990s, schedule II opioid analgesics were primarily used in operating rooms and inpatient settings, since they needed to be administered intravenously (IV) or intramuscularly (IM). During the 1990s several new extended-release formulas of existing prescription opioids were developed and approved for marketing. These drugs provided patients in pain with the ability to achieve sustained pain relief that did not require an IV or IM infusion (Woolf and Hashmi 2004).

Much attention has been given to the dramatically increased rates of OxyContin and hydrocodone (usually as Vicodin) abuse that followed the increased use of these drugs for pain relief. As mentioned earlier, several factors led to a significant increase in the prescribing of all prescription opiates during the 1990s. Results of several epidemiological studies indicate a high prevalence of lifetime abuse of other substances, and of substance-related disorders in patients with OxyContin dependence, suggesting that substance abuse predated the use of OxyContin (e.g., Potter et al. 2004). Several aspects of OxyContin made it almost uniquely desirable as a drug of abuse, which will be described in chapter 8.

Development of Iatrogenic Addiction

The addiction of a patient to a drug initially prescribed for a medical condition is referred to as an *iatrogenic* addiction. Opioid prescribing falls into two major subgroups: (1) treatment of acute pain with short-term opioids, and (2) treatment of chronic pain with long-term opioids. Although addiction is rare with short-term use, long-term administration of opioids results in opiate abuse or dependence in 2.8% to 18.9% of patients—corresponding with rates of opioid abuse or addiction in the general population (Compton and Volkow 2006).

A couple of recent studies looked at prescription opioids as the source of iatrogenic addiction. One study by Fishbain and colleagues (2008) found that chronic prescription opioid use will lead to abuse/addiction in a small percentage of chronic pain patients, but a larger percentage will demonstrate aberrant drug-related behavior (behaviors such as requesting early refills or borrowing medications from family or friends) and illicit drug use. These percentages drop significantly if the chronic pain patients are screened for current or past history of alcohol or drug abuse. Another study using a nationally representative survey examined the rates of opioid and other drug abuse in patients receiving prescription opioids for chronic noncancer pain. Users of prescribed opioids experienced higher rates of opioid and nonopioid abuse compared with people who did not use prescribed opioids, but these higher rates were partially explained by the presence of depressive and anxiety disorders. The authors concluded that their results were consistent with previous findings that psychiatric illness led to higher rates of iatrogenic abuse and dependency among prescription opioid users than is found in prescription opioid users who do not have psychiatric illness (Edlund et al. 2007).

Several validated screening questionnaires, such as the Opioid Risk Tool (Webster and Webster 2005) and the Revised Screener and Opioid Assessment for Patients with Pain (Butler et al. 2008), are now available to help physicians identify patients at risk of developing an iatrogenic addiction to prescription painkillers. These screens typically identify the patient's level of risk as low, moderate, or high (Butler et al. 2008; Butler et al. 2007; Webster and Webster 2005). This risk placement, especially when used with behavioral observations of the patient by the physician or other staff (see table 5.1), allows the physician to improve care by providing appropriate structure to the therapy and monitoring of the patient; it also helps physicians identify patients who may need consultation with a pain specialist or an addiction specialist (Argoff and Silvershein 2009). Also, research suggests that patients with a history of substance abuse receiving prescription opioids benefit from actively participating in their recovery while taking the opioid (Ling, Wesson, and Smith 2005). These efforts are essential; however, many people with a history of substance use will not divulge this information to caregivers, and it is very difficult to diagnose addiction in a pain population, requiring a level of expertise in both pain and addiction that is difficult to find.

Table 5.1

Risk Assessment of Patient Behavior during Prescription Opioid Therapy

More suggestive of addiction*	Less suggestive of addiction
• Concurrent abuse of alcohol or illicit drugs	• Aggressive complaining about the need for more drugs
• Declining ability to function at work, in the family, or socially that appears to be related to drug use	• Drug hoarding during periods of reduced symptoms
• Injecting oral formulations	• Openly acquiring similar drugs from other medical sources
• Multiple-dose escalations or other nonadherence with therapy despite warnings	• Requesting specific drugs
• Obtaining prescription drugs from nonmedical sources	• Reporting psychic effects not intended by the physician
• Prescription forgery	• Resistance to a change in therapy associated with tolerable negative effects accompanied by anxiety related to the return of severe symptoms
• Repeated resistance to changes in therapy despite obvious drug-related negative physical or psychological effects	• Unapproved use of the drug to treat another symptom
• Repeatedly seeking prescriptions from other physicians or emergency departments without informing prescriber	• Unsanctioned dose escalation or other nonadherence with therapy on one or two occasions
• Selling prescription drugs	
• Stealing or borrowing drugs from others	

(Passik 2009)   * *Documented in patient's medical chart.*

One way to determine whether pain control is adequate is to consider whether the use of added opioids has resulted in improvements in the functioning, physical ability, psychological well-being, family and other social interactions, and health care resource use compared with unwanted effects such as daytime sedation, mental confusion, and constipation. Although a pattern of abnormal behavior may be grounds for caution, a history of opioid abuse need not necessarily exclude a patient from treatment with an opioid (Ling, Wesson, and Smith 2005).

The appropriate prescribing of opioids for pain is relatively easy when treating acute pain, such as a broken leg. The treatment of chronic pain is much more difficult, not well studied, and fraught with secondary psychological issues. Physicians want to relieve pain and suffering, but opioids may not be a reasonable choice for treatment of some chronic pain. The jury is out, and problems continue to multiply as we expose more people to long-term opioid therapy.

More Research Needed

Opioids act much like any addictive substance to increase dopamine and activate the reward center of the brain. As we learn more about the neurobiology of addiction, we better recognize addiction as a disease and understand the confounding behaviors that define active addiction in our families and communities. Increased medical use of these powerful substances puts more people at risk of becoming addicted to opioids. Without adequate information, lacking substantial medical research about treatment of chronic pain with opioids, physicians continue to prescribe these medications at alarming rates. They are tremendous pain relievers; however, they are highly rewarding and remarkably addictive. More research is needed to guide appropriate decision making for those suffering from chronic pain and to limit the risk of addiction.

CHAPTER 6

How Opioids Are Abused

Opioids are available for use orally, anally, by intramuscular injection, sublingually (under the tongue), and as patches that allow medicine to be absorbed through the skin. When using opioids to get high, people want to experience the drug's effects immediately. As a result, they will use the drugs in ways they are not intended. Use can differ by preferences, as some people refuse to inject or smoke drugs. The government and the pharmaceutical industry have tried various methods to limit and prevent abuse of prescribed opioids, with varying results. This chapter examines differing methods for using prescribed opioids in an abusive manner.

The *pharmacokinetics* of a drug describes the rate at which the drug is absorbed into the body, distributed throughout the body, metabolized, and eliminated from the body. The abuse potential of a drug is partially dependent on the pharmacokinetic profile of the drug. Factors that affect drug pharmacokinetics include the chosen route of administration, how much of the drug is administered, and the rate of onset of its effects (Farre and Cami 1991). The route of administration is the factor most likely to be modified by drug abusers to increase the drug's intensity, and also represents the primary target of abuse deterrent formulations or ADFs (Budman, Serrano, and Butler 2009).

The time it takes the drug to reach the brain varies with different routes of administration. Routes of administration that facilitate a faster delivery of the drug to the brain seem to be associated with greater abuse potential; this is true because a more rapid rise in blood plasma concentration of an addictive drug produces greater drug liking and reinforcement than a slower rise in blood plasma concentration of the drug (Mansbach and Moore 2006). For example, crack cocaine, a smoked form of cocaine, is considered more addicting than snorted cocaine because it reaches the brain so much faster. For most drugs, including opioids, routes of administration can be ranked, from the fastest delivery to the brain to the slowest, as follows: inhalation by smoking, intravenous, intranasal, and oral ingestion (Oldendorf 1992). The same principle applies to drugs that are more rapidly absorbed into the blood and brain. These drugs have a higher potential for abuse than similar drugs that are absorbed more slowly because they produce a greater "rush." Examples include pentobarbital among the barbiturates, diazepam among the benzodiazepines, and morphine among the opiates (Mansbach and Moore 2006; deWit, Bodker, and Ambre 1992; deWit, Dudish, and Ambre 1993). Thus, psychoactive drugs are more highly reinforcing to people predisposed to addiction if the drug has a rapid onset of effect, higher potency, briefer duration of action, high purity, water solubility (for intravenous use), or high volatility (ability to vaporize if smoked) (Longo et al. 2000). Studies evaluating the abuse liability of various opioid medications clearly indicate that controlled-release formulations, such as MS-Contin, and agents with a long half-life, such as methadone and levo-alpha acetyl methadol (LAAM), have lower abuse potential and less street value than high-peaking, rapid-onset opioid formulations, such as OxyContin (once the formulation is tampered) (Brookoff 1993).

Interestingly, the abuse potential of prescription opioids may be unrelated to their painkilling ability. A study examining the relative abuse potential and analgesic potency of oral oxycodone (10, 20, and 40 mg), hydrocodone (15, 30, and 45 mg), and hydromorphone (10, 17.5, and 25 mg) found that the abuse liability profile and relative potency of these three commonly used opioids do not differ substantially from one another and suggest that analgesic potency may be a poor predictor of the abuse potential of pre-scription opioids (Walsh et al. 2008).

Factors Influencing Choice of Route of Administration

Abuse of prescription opioids can involve altering the intended route of administration to intensify the desired drug effect. Several factors influence the route of administration that is chosen by abusers of prescription opioids. These include the drug formulation, drug availability, the course of an individual's drug abuse history, the social environment of the user, and the availability of information on how to tamper with a drug for alternate routes of administration. These factors appear to be strongly intercon-nected (Budman, Serrano, and Butler 2009).

Methods Used to Alter the Route of Administration of Prescription Opioids

All prescription opioids (except for pure antagonists such as naloxone) have at least some potential for abuse. The following pages describe techniques used to tamper with various prescription opioids in order to achieve a more intense effect than ingesting the unaltered drug can provide. Some of these depictions were found in the published literature, while others were obtained directly from the Internet. The descriptions on the Internet are remarkably effective and up-to-date. On some sites they appear to be written by people with substantial pharmacological expertise.

Buprenorphine

Buprenorphine is used for detoxification of opioids and for maintenance treatment of opioid addiction. It is a partial opioid agonist and can be used for intoxication. Buprenorphine comes in three forms:

- Buprenex is for intramuscular and intravenous injection to treat moderate pain.
- Subutex is a sublingual tablet for the treatment of opioid addiction, primarily used in structured settings.

• Suboxone, also used for the treatment of opioid addiction, is a combination of buprenorphine and naloxone. Naloxone, an opioid antagonist or opioid receptor blocker, is added to Suboxone to prevent intravenous use of the medication. If injected, it causes sudden, severe opioid withdrawal rather than intoxication.

Chua and Lee (2006) presented two cases of buprenorphine abuse, one by an addict who ground up his Subutex with midazolam, a potent benzodiazepine, and used it intravenously instead of taking it orally, and the other case by an addict who had been injecting Subutex IV. A user on Erowid.org described a method of grinding up a buprenorphine formulation and placing it rectally:

Mixed 15ml h20 and 2mg powdered suboxone into a syringe (no needle). Lubed it up and aspirated it rectally. Onset was about 20 min. Felt extremely relaxed. 60 min after dosing I got a mild euphoria and sedation. Felt pretty good compared to my usual dose which is only about .25 2x a day. The increase in dose may skew the results. A few hours later and I feel pretty good. Overall I think I'd much rather snort it just because of the prep involved plugging it. I would only do this when I'm bored with my basic sub routine and have some to spare.

On a side note. I find it much harder to quit subs compared to OC or heroin. Withdrawal is extremely drawn out and intense. I feel like I'm stuck with the crappy orange tasting pills for awhile because I can't afford to ride out the withdrawal for a few weeks. At least they don't show up on a standard 5 panel drug test.

Codeine

There are legitimate concerns over the recreational use of codeine that is formulated with other active ingredients such as acetaminophen (potential liver damage), aspirin (gastrointestinal bleeding), caffeine, and ibuprofen. Many people who abuse or use codeine nonmedically believe the pharmaceutical companies combine codeine with other drugs such as acetaminophen to prevent excessive use (Cone 2006). Codeine is available over the counter (without a prescription) in Canada and Mexico.

Users concerned over toxicity from ingesting the large amounts of acetaminophen and aspirin frequently contained in these codeine formulations can now simply access the Internet to find recipes on how to "purify" the formulation. A variety of "cold-water extraction" recipes describe this extraction method.

A brief description of the method from Erowid.org is as follows: ". . . you can dissolve 20 tablets in 50 ml of hot water, cool the water down to 10C, filter the solution and end up with the same amount of codeine as the tablets contained but only a fraction of the original amount of A/A." Of interest is that a fairly weak opioid, like codeine, has its following in spite of the availability of so many more powerful opioids.

"Loads" (Doriden and Codeine)

"Loads" is a combination of the sedative drug glutethimide (Doriden) and codeine. Loads emerged in the illicit street drug market of Los Angeles in the early 1980s as a heroin substitute. This drug combination produces an intense state of intoxication. Frequent use can lead to a serious and complicated withdrawal process because the user experiences both sedative and opioid withdrawal. Glutethimide is rarely prescribed in the United States.

One load contains two tablets of glutethimide and four tablets of codeine. Some users state the high from loads is better than the high from heroin, and one study of sixty patients admitted to a hospital to detoxify from loads found that most of the patients had switched from heroin to loads (Khajawall, Sramek, and Simpson 1982). Although the typical IV "rush" (or sudden onset) is absent, this desired effect of IV heroin can be mimicked somewhat by taking loads on an empty stomach. Ingestion of alcohol reportedly intensifies this rush, suggesting an increase in the rate of drug absorption. Many of the patients in the Khajawall study stated that they encountered significant problems while taking loads, such as coma, convulsions, peripheral neuropathies, major automobile crashes, cuts, and burns. The attractiveness of loads over heroin may be explained by the potent enzyme-inducing property of glutethimide that converts a higher amount of the codeine to morphine than occurs without it. Thus, glutethimide has the ability to transform codeine, a normally minimally abused opioid with a high side-effect profile and low affinity for opioid receptors, into a more potent mu-opioid agonist (Khajawall, Sramek, and Simpson 1982).

Fentanyl Transdermal Patches (Duragesic)

Fentanyl patches, even after they are used and discarded by a pain patient, may contain lethal amounts of residual drug (Tharp, Winecker, and Winston 2004). On a theoretical basis, approximately 28% of the total fentanyl dose (up to 2.8 mg for the highest dose) should remain in the patch following use for the recommended three days (Cone 2006).

Abusers may resort to unusual means of obtaining used patches, such as removing the patches from elderly nursing home residents (*Columbia Daily Tribune* 2002) and deceased individuals (Flannagan, Butts, and Anderson 1996), and searching hospital and nursing home dumpsters for discarded patches (Cone 2006).

The properties of fentanyl—including its stability, potency, and ease in which it penetrates the blood-brain barrier—make it amenable to misuse by numerous routes of administration. Drug users administer fentanyl from the patch by applying it to various body regions and also by chewing, sucking, and vaginally inserting the patch. Some users attempt to increase the speed of absorption of fentanyl from the patch by applying a heat source such as a heating pad over the patch or by soaking in a hot tub. Methods for removing the fentanyl from the patch include squeezing the fentanyl gel out of the patch, removing it with a syringe, and extracting it with various solvents. Extracted fentanyl has been eaten, injected, or smoked in a glass pipe, vaporized on aluminum foil, or added to a cigarette. A Department of Justice Internet site (DEA 2004) states that "patches have also been frozen, cut into pieces and placed under the tongue or in the cheek cavity for drug absorption through the oral mucosa."

The following descriptions of user experiences in fentanyl tampering were posted on Erowid.org:

#1: This time I cut open the patch and squeezed most of the gel out into a little ball, and smoked a large portion of it, ignoring all the rumors of how dangerous and lethal that could be. It turned out that the high was that of oxycontin, but without the euphoric mental effects.

#2: Before I use my [Actiq lozenge] I do a mouthwash rinse and brush my mouth with Straight Baking Soda, Arm and Hammer works great. Afterward I rinse and then suck on Lozenge to moisten it up. Then I apply the Lozenge directly into a bag/box of baking soda and get a nice coating, then stick the thing in my mouth against my cheek. This somehow increases the bioavailability of the drug matrix into the blood stream by the chemical action/reaction of the baking soda. I can increase the effects and longevity of the Lozenge by almost 30–40%. This is great for those of us who are on strict regiments and contracts of limited meds.

#3: The smallest [D]uragesic patches are 25/ug per hour rclcase 1.8mg over three days before they are changed for a fresh patch. This actually theoretically leaves .7 mg of fentanyl in the spent patches. Fentanyl being soluble in alcohol, the spent patches were cut up in small pieces and soaked in a small amount of 99% anhydrous isopropyl alcohol (70% would probably work too). After some time, overnight or even weeks as the spent patches were simply added to the jar, the alcohol was filtered and the filter expressed so as much of the substance would fall in a glass dish. Basil leaf or some other smokable herb was placed in the alcohol and the alcohol was allowed to evaporate. The herb was smeared and even a razor used to scrape up any residue to place it on the herb.

This fentanyl-laced herb was smoked for strong opiate effect. The amount of herb used determines potency, more patches and less herb obviously makes it more potent. One or two hits would produce not a rush but a definite floating feeling with colorful CEV's [closed eye visuals]. Standing up assured one was very intoxicating as one felt wobbly. After a few small bowls, sweat would appear on the forehead and one certainly felt "loaded" for a few hours.

Morphine Preparations

Morphine misuse occurs by many routes of administration. Immediate-release formulations are administered primarily by the oral, intranasal, IV, and smoked routes. One user reported a method for converting morphine sulfate into heroin (diacetylmorphine) for IV use (Cone 2006). Misuse of the extended-release formulations occurs primarily by the oral and intranasal routes. Attempts to render the controlled-release formulation into a form suitable for IV use appear to be difficult without special processing. For example, one user reported, "These are time-release tablets with a plastic-like coating and a wax binder matrix inside that is not water-soluble. It forms a gum if cooked up and will clog a syringe as it cools" (Cone 2006). Several methods to circumvent this problem have been reported.

A user on Erowid.org describes the process of converting morphine tablets into a form suitable for ingestion through alternate routes:

After my experiences with snorting crushed up morphine sulfate pills, which were quite disappointing, I asked a friend why nothing really had happened. He told me snorting sulfate salts doesn't work well, since sulfates aren't that good water-soluble and I should change the morphine sulfate to morphine hcl, which is suitable for snorting.

(I checked that solubility matter and it turned out that morphine sulfate is even better soluble in water than the hydrochloride. . . . So to be honest, I have no clue why the crushed pills did barely anything good. Lately I tried them again and they worked just as fine as the hcl.)

I did so and ended up with about 300 mg of pure morphine hcl powder. I divided the powder in 15 parts, 20 mg each and snorted one of those little bumps. First thing I felt was a burning sensation in my nose, worse than that you get from meth. I was waiting for the effects to begin, but nothing really happened and I was getting disappointed, but then suddenly after 10 mins the effects started to kick in.

This gave me a really nice feeling, that typical opiate high. You get relaxed, a little bit euphoric and don't care about nothing. I just sat down, read some magazines, listened to music and watched TV. I snorted the first bump at about 8 pm and at 10:30 pm I decided to do another little bump to intensify the feelings. I divided one of the 20 mg bumps in two and snorted that. This time there were [sic] absolutely no pain, I wonder why? :) I continued reading, listening to music and watching TV for a few hours until 3 am. Then I went to bed, had that dreamlike state I use to get when trying to sleep on opiates and finally felt asleep at 5 a.m.

The conclusion is, that when you come across some morphine pills, which all are morphine sf, extract the morphine, change it to the HCl salt and snort it. Eating is a terrible waste (I need 80 mg oral, but only 30 mg nasal) so if you're not into IV'ing snort it. [The user then provided the instructions for extracting the morphine.]

Methadone

In methadone clinics, methadone is dispensed in prepared individual doses and is mixed with fruit juice to discourage IV use. There are anecdotes of individuals receiving liquid methadone in methadone clinics and pretending to swallow the dose in front of clinic staff but actually spitting out the liquid dose outside the clinic for resale.

Pentazocine (Talwin)

In the 1970s and early 1980s, Talwin was combined with the blue-colored antihistamine tablet tripelennamine and used intravenously, a combination known on the street as "Ts and Blues"(see page 134) (Ling, Wesson, and Smith 2005).

Oxycodone (Percodan, Percocet, OxyContin)

The oxycodone content of OxyContin ranges from 10 mg to 80 mg. When taken orally, OxyContin tablets release oxycodone over a twelve-hour period; however, when the controlled-release mechanism is destroyed by crushing the tablet, the oxycodone can be snorted, ingested, or injected, and it is this large delivery of the active drug in a relatively brief time period, relative to the intact OxyContin tablet and the low-dose immediate-release form, that makes the OxyContin formulation of oxycodone highly sought after (Ling, Wesson, and Smith 2005). Percodan and Percocet were the oxycodone medications available prior to OxyContin and they have 10 mg or less of oxycodone. The high doses of OxyContin were a dramatic shift in oral opioid dosing, using large amounts in a single tablet. At one time 160-mg OxyContin tablets were available; now the largest is 80 mg. The large doses also added to the desirability of OxyContin on the street.

Although abuse of oxycodone appears to be primarily via the oral route, many users seem to prefer the intranasal route. One user reported that "snorting" a crushed 40-mg time-release oxycodone tablet produced effects in four minutes, compared with more than twenty minutes with chewing and swallowing. Another user reported: "At first we would just swallow the wonderful little pill . . . but 1 day we decided to experiment with it, so we crushed up the pill and sniffed it. We were shocked, the effects of

sniffing oxycontin are way more intense than swallowing it. Within 2 min
it started working" (Cone 2006).

Some users report IV ingestion of oxycodone. An IV user offered the
following comments regarding his experience: "I cooked up a pill and shot
it into my vein. It was the best high I had ever had. The intensity of the
come-up was so great that after 10 seconds I could not even stand up. I just
laid on my bed in total and complete bliss. So from then on every time I
got oxy I injected it. I was starting to do damage to my veins, and I could
see the scar tissue protruding from the skin. My friends, who do not even
smoke pot got very worried about me, so I quit oxy all together. I stopped
injecting and the wounds healed. I did not suffer withdrawal but I felt
something was gone out of my life" (Cone 2006).

The IV use of time-release preparations of oxycodone requires a degree
of ingenuity in separating the drug from the coating and other "waxy"
components. One method involves scraping off the coating, crushing
the pill, heating it in a spoon with water, adding cold water (which hardens
the wax), and filtering the solution through cotton into a syringe. The cold-
water extraction method used to isolate codeine from other constituents
in the pill (described earlier) is also reported to work for oxycodone
(Cone 2006).

The following description of a user experience with OxyContin (OC)
tampering was posted on Erowid.org:

> I guess I'll start with the preparations. Mindset and setting are not so
> much a factor, as after smoking OC you will be euphoric and high as hell.
> The only thing to keep in mind is that the smell is pretty distinct and
> pungent, so it's probably a good idea to be somewhere "cool," but that
> goes without saying.
>
> The effects will come on in 5 minutes or less, and are almost identical
> to oral or nasal administration, except I have found them to be more
> powerful, and less addicting. In prior experiences with insufflation
> [nasal inhalation of powder] the next days I would have an insane desire

to just keep buying and putting the stuff up my nose. With smoking however, the next day the thoughts about doing it are far less intense. I would highly recommend at least trying this method if you are someone who has access to OC.

Hydrocodone (Vicodin)

The following descriptions of user experiences with hydrocodone tampering were posted on Erowid.org:

> I am aware that regular Acetaminophen doses are extremely hard on the liver, so for about the last 4 or so months I've been using a cold water extraction technique to alleviate this problem when I'm dosing with Hydrocodone.
>
> I enjoy dosing this way more then [sic] any other way due to a couple of factors. 1. It's safer and healthier. 2. In liquid form opiates tend to hit (effect) [sic] me much more quickly. The only really downside to this method is the taste of the liquid, it's terribly bitter. To counteract this I have used Crystal Light or Stevia (a natural sweetener found at most health food stores).

Hydrocodone is readily available to health care personnel (doctors and nurses), who sometimes use it and become addicted. They develop rapid tolerance and may begin to take it by the handful. Treatment centers have reported admitting doctors who are taking up to 100 Vicodin tablets per day. Surprisingly, there appears to be tolerance to the liver damage caused by the high dose of acetaminophen that is ingested. Liver damage is occasionally noted with high-dose Vicodin use, but regularly there is none to be found.

Hydromorphone (Dilaudid)

A user on Erowid.org described how he altered hydromorphone into a preparation suitable for IV use:

The inhalation (snorting) route didn't cause any great rush of sensation—it was more subtle. But the IV route produced an incredible rush—feelings of warmth, well being, very mild sedation and that hard to describe but wonderful "body buzz." It took only about two minutes to fully set in and after having a cigarette I felt "just capitol." HM 2mg tablets are tiny and contain no acetaminophen (AM). When crushed very finely and thoroughly 2 x 2mg tabs easily dissolve in 1 CC of hot (but not boiling water). Injection procedure and hygiene are critical. I once ended up with a cellulitis (abscess) on my ankle from bad hygiene that could have killed me (I used a syringe multiple times at the same site). It had to be lanced at the hospital and I was in severe pain for weeks with an ankle the size of a football. Needless to say I won't repeat that foolish mistake again. I'm now very careful and will illustrate that. I'm by no means saying this is something you should do—remember that IV is always a dangerous practice.

Abuse-Deterrent Prescription Opioid Formulations

Given the abuse potential of prescription opioids and the relative ease in altering the route of administration to obtain a more intense high, pressure has been growing on pharmaceutical companies to develop prescription opioid formulations that deter abuse yet remain readily accessible for pain management (Budman, Serrano, and Butler 2009).

An example of the successful development of an abuse-deterrent formulation is the case of pentazocine (Talwin). Talwin was first marketed in 1967, and during the 1970s became widely abused by physicians and other health care personnel because of its placement outside the strict DEA schedule II monitoring system and by the belief that it was nonaddictive. The preferred method of Talwin abuse was intravenous use in combination with the antihistamine tripelennamine, known as "Ts and Blues." At one point Talwin abuse was so rampant, especially in the Midwest, that the manufacturer contemplated removing the drug from the market. Talwin was ultimately reformulated to include the opioid antagonist naloxone (Talwin Nx). When Talwin Nx is taken as directed, the user experiences only the pentazocine effect because of poor oral naloxone absorption, but if the tablet is injected, the naloxone blocks the opioid effects of the pentazocine and precipitates acute opioid withdrawal. This reformulation of Talwin resulted in a dramatic decrease in the abuse of Ts and Blues (Ling, Wesson, and Smith 2005).

Although abuse deterrence was not the primary goal, the controlled-release formulations of oxycodone, morphine, and Dilaudid were expected to reduce the potential of abuse by delaying the rate at which the active drug entered the bloodstream, crossed the blood-brain barrier into the brain, and occupied opioid receptors. The "rush" and euphoria that come from high concentrations of an opioid rapidly entering the brain did not occur with these new formulations, which were thought to discourage abuse. However, many opioid abusers figured out how to circumvent the time-release mechanism to accelerate the drug's entry into the brain and achieve a more intense euphoria and high from the large amount of oxycodone contained in the OxyContin tablet. The simple act of crushing and then swallowing, snorting, or injecting the pill achieved this end (Sproule et al. 2009).

The alteration of prescription opioids involves an attempt by abusers to manipulate the drug to make the active ingredient immediately available (especially for extended-release formulations) in a form conducive to use via alternate routes of administration. Various abuse deterrent formulations (ADFs) are now in development, each with a unique mechanism to thwart this behavior. These include formulations with physical barriers resistant to common methods of tampering, such as crushing the pill and extracting the active ingredient, with the goal of preventing abuse through intravenous, snorting, and chewing routes of administration (Katz 2008); and antagonist-agonist combinations that contain an opioid antagonist that blocks the opioid effect if the pill was tampered with (Sunshine et al. 1988). Although ADFs may prevent abuse through alternate routes of administration, they will probably have little to no impact on those who prefer to abuse these drugs by taking the drug intact (Budman, Serrano, and Butler. 2009; Webster, Bath, and Medve 2009). As soon as ADFs are made available, online sites explain how to extract the pure opioid, so these formulations may prevent simple acts to change the route of administration, but motivated opioid users will find a way to get the drug in the form they want it.

Other ADFs include the use of *prodrugs,* which have to be metabolized to an active form after ingestion to produce a pharmacological effect, as well as ADFs that incorporate an aversive stimulus, such as niacin or capsaicin, which produces an uncomfortable physical sensation if the product is tampered with before ingestion (Katz 2008). The impact of these ADFs will probably not be seen until most prescription opioid analgesics are ADFs (Budman, Serrano, and Butler 2009; Passik 2009).

A novel approach intended to deter or greatly reduce the abuse of OxyContin was recently introduced by Purdue Pharma. On September 24, 2009, an FDA advisory panel approved a new formulation of oxycodone hydrochloride (OxyContin) that is more difficult to crush or dissolve, and that may deter abuse of the product. Although there is no proof that the new formulation is safer, the panel agreed that making the pills harder to crush, chew, or dissolve into liquid may deter abusers. When the new version of the drug is dissolved in water, it produces a gel, which makes attempting to snort or inject the drug more difficult. In one lab test, Purdue researchers used sixteen different household tools to try to crush the tablet into small particles. All sixteen tools easily crushed the original OxyContin tablets to a fine powder, and although four of the tools managed to break down the new tablet into shavings or particles, none could break it down any further into powder. The FDA is not required to follow the advice of its advisory committees, but it usually does. However, FDA staff reviewers conceded that the technology will probably not make a substantial difference in the overall abuse potential of OxyContin (Hitt 2009).

In addition to the development of ADFs, the development of new pain medications or formulations with minimal abuse potential will be a vitally important strategy to combat or reduce the current epidemic of prescription opioid abuse. Compounds that act on a combination of opioid receptors, such as mu and delta, are likely to provide powerful pain relief without producing tolerance or dependence (Manchikanti 2006). Research is working to develop non-opioid, nonaddicting treatments of chronic pain, limiting the need for opioids, which will decrease access and abuse. This may be the most effective means of ending the opioid epidemic.

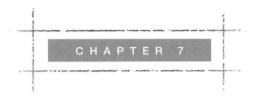

Opioid Pharmacology
and the Individual Opioids

Opioids have been the mainstay of pain treatment for thousands of years, and they remain so today. Opioids such as morphine work by mimicking the actions of naturally occurring opioids in the brain. These brain chemicals are referred to as the endogenous (produced in the body) opioid peptides (Gutstein and Akil 2006). Although a multitude of newer opioids have been developed with pharmacological properties that are similar to morphine, morphine remains the gold standard against which the effectiveness of all new painkillers is measured (Gutstein and Akil 2006).

Opioid medications produce their diverse biological effects by binding to opioid receptors that are distributed throughout the brain and body. When these drugs bind to the opioid receptors, the receptors transmit chemical signals through various intracellular signaling pathways that results in the drug's effect (Fiellin, Friedland, and Gourevitch 2006). The opioid medications and the endogenous opioids both bind to the same opioid receptors; the difference is that opioid medications, in essence, overstimulate a natural, internal opioid system and produce a far more powerful effect. Most, but not all, prescription opioids are opioid agonists—they fully activate the opioid receptor when they bind to it. The opposite of an agonist is an antagonist, which is a drug that blocks the activity of the receptor it binds to (like naloxone and naltrexone).

Four Groups of Opioid Medications

Opioid medications can be placed into four groups, based on their activity at the opioid receptor site where they bind to produce their effect. The first group consists of drugs that bind to and activate opioid receptors in the brain, the agonists. It includes the natural opium derivatives morphine and codeine, the semisynthetic opioid derivatives such as hydromorphone (Dilaudid), oxymorphone (Numorphan), hydrocodone (Vicodin and others), oxycodone (OxyContin, Percocet, and others), and the synthetic opioids such as meperidine (Demerol), fentanyl (Sublimaze, Duragesic), methadone, and propoxyphene (Darvocet, Darvon).

The second group includes opioids that bind to multiple opioid receptors in the brain, where they activate certain opioid receptor types and block the actions of others. These drugs are referred to as mixed agonist-antagonists, and include pentazocine (Talwin), nalbuphine (Nubain), and butorphanol (Stadol). They are not as effective for pain relief as the pure opioid agonists.

Opioids in the third group are referred to as partial agonists because they bind to and activate opioid receptors, although to a lesser extent than a pure agonist such as morphine. These do not fully stimulate the mu-opioid receptor and have a "ceiling effect"; the pain relief or high derived from the medicine tops out at a certain level, unlike pure opioid agonists. Drugs in this class include buprenorphine (Buprenex, Subutex, and Suboxone) (Armstrong and Cozza 2003).

Medications in the fourth group are referred to as opioid antagonists because they bind to opioid receptors and fully block their activity. This class includes naltrexone and naloxone. Naloxone and naltrexone block the effects of opioid agonists (like morphine, oxycodone, and heroin) and in the process "evict" the molecule of the agonist drug. Naloxone is given to people who have overdosed on opioids to block the opioid's toxic effects in an attempt to save their lives. People who are unable to breathe and appear to be comatose from an opioid overdose may wake up and talk within minutes of a naloxone injection.

Recently, laboratory research and clinical trials have shown an unexpected, paradoxical effect of these opioid antagonist drugs in enhancing rather than undermining the pain-relieving effects of opioids such as morphine in the treatment of breakthrough post-operative pain and severe intractable pain. There is also evidence that drugs in this group are capable of producing analgesia when used alone in conditions such as Crohn's disease, irritable bowel syndrome, and fibromyalgia (Leavitt 2009). This is new, inconclusive research and these medications are not approved or regularly used for these purposes.

In addition to being grouped according to their action at the opioid receptor, opioid drugs can also be grouped according to their chemical class. The four chemical classes of opioids are as follows (Trescot et al. 2008):

- Phenanthrenes are the prototypical opioids. Opioids in this group include morphine, codeine, hydromorphone, levorphanol, oxycodone, hydrocodone, oxymorphone, buprenorphine, nalbuphine, and butorphanol.
- Benzomorphans: pentazocine is the only member of this class.
- Phenylpiperidines include fentanyl, alfentanil, sufentanil, and meperidine.
- Diphenylheptanes include propoxyphene and methadone.

The Pharmacology of Opioid Drugs

Opium comes from the unripe seed capsules of the poppy plant, *Papaver somniferum*. Although raw opium contains numerous alkaloids, only a few such as morphine, codeine, thebaine, and papaverine have an identified use in medicine. Because morphine synthesis is difficult, the medications are still obtained primarily from opium (Gutstein and Akil 2006).

Numerous opioid medications are synthetic derivatives of morphine and thebaine, which are produced by relatively simple modifications of the parent molecule. Examples of this include transforming morphine into codeine by methyl substitution on the phenolic hydroxyl group; the transformation of morphine to diacetylmorphine by acetylation at the 3 and 6 positions (to produce heroin); and the transformation of morphine into hydromorphine, oxymorphone, hydrocodone, and oxycodone.

Endogenous Opioid Peptides

The endogenous opioid system is the internal system of opioid receptors and opioid-like chemical messengers that are important to physiologic functioning throughout the brain and body. The endogenous opioid system is complex. It carries out many diverse functions, including a sensory role that helps block pain; a role in helping to regulate the functioning of gastrointestinal, endocrine, and autonomic systems; an emotional role as the origin of the powerful, rewarding, and potentially addicting effects of opioids; and a cognitive role that is involved in regulating learning and memory (Gutstein and Akil 2006). When something produces pain, the endogenous opioids are released and bind to the opioid receptors to stimulate their action in an attempt to limit the sensation of pain. When stimulated, they send a series of chemical messages to different parts of the brain and body that reduce the pain response (Trescot et al. 2008).

Opioid Receptors

The three major types of opioid receptors are *mu, kappa,* and *delta* receptors, and they are found throughout the brain, spinal cord, and peripheral nervous systems. They are plentiful in the central respiratory centers, which control breathing (Pharo and Zhou 2005; White and Irvine 1999). Opioid drugs produce their diverse biological effects by binding to these three different opioid receptors. When this happens, the receptors transmit chemical signals through various intracellular signaling pathways (Fiellin, Friedland, and Gourevitch 2006). The three primary opiate receptors and their Greek symbols, their location in the brain, and the functions that they activate when stimulated include the following (Trescot et al. 2008):

Mu (μ): Mu receptors are found primarily in the brain stem and the medial thalamus. Mu receptor activity is responsible for supraspinal analgesia (pain relief sensed in the brain), respiratory depression, euphoria, sedation, decreased movement in the stomach and intestines, and intoxication associated with physical dependence.

Kappa (κ): Kappa receptors are found in the limbic and other diencephalic areas of the brain, brain stem, and spinal cord.

They are responsible for spinal analgesia (pain relief experienced at the level of the spinal cord), sedation, difficulty breathing, dependence, and dysphoria.

Delta (δ): Delta receptors are largely confined to the brain and their effects are not well understood. They may be responsible for psychotic and dysphoric effects.

The major opioid receptor associated with pain relief is the mu receptor. All pain-relieving opioids stimulate the mu receptor and all opioids that are addicting do the same. There is a high degree of similarity between the opioid drugs that have been used for pain relief for centuries, such as morphine, and the more recently developed opioid painkillers, like fentanyl. They all act the same way, as mu receptor agonists.

Absorption and Distribution

Opioid drugs are usually absorbed quickly from the gastrointestinal tract, although most opioids, including morphine, are partially broken down in the liver—called hepatic first-pass metabolism—before they enter the brain. This process reduces the amount of drug that reaches the brain. Most opioids rapidly produce their effects when taken intravenously. However, opioids, as well as all other drugs, have to pass through a protective barrier before they enter the brain. This barrier is called the blood-brain barrier, and because a large portion of the brain is composed of fat, opioid drugs that are quicker at penetrating fatty tissue (fat-soluble) have a shorter time from ingestion to action. Morphine crosses the blood-brain barrier at a much slower rate than opioids that are more fat-soluble such as codeine, heroin, and methadone (Gutstein and Akil 2006).

The Individual Opioids

In addition to opium, which is found in nature, the pharmaceutical industry has created more than twenty prescription opioids that have received FDA approval for sale in the United States and are primarily used for pain relief. Most of these drugs have a potential for abuse, and the federal Drug Enforcement Administration (DEA) and state agencies attempt to restrict these drugs (Simoni-Wastila and Strickler 2004). Only DEA-licensed physicians can prescribe these drugs, and physicians and pharmacists can be arrested and imprisoned for illicit prescribing and for not controlling or cutting off patients who divert or sell their prescriptions (Longo et al. 2000). Table 7.1 summarizes the prescription opioids available in the United States (see pages 162–164).

Opioids of Natural Origin

Opium

The opium poppy plant, *Papaver somniferum,* was grown in the Mediterranean region as early as 5000 BCE and has since been cultivated in a number of regions throughout the world. Opium is obtained by slitting the unripe seedpod of the poppy plant and drying the milky fluid in the sun. The extract may be used in liquid, solid, or powder form. A more modern method of harvesting opium is by extracting the opiate compounds from the mature dried plant through a process known as the *industrial poppy straw* process. More than 500 tons of opium or equivalents in poppy straw concentrate are legally imported into the United States each year for legitimate medical use (DEA 2005). Although opium is still used in the form of paregoric to treat diarrhea, most opium imported into the United States is further broken down into its constituents. Termed alkaloids, the constituents obtained from opium are divided into two distinct chemical classes, the phenanthrenes and the benzylisoquinolines. The principal phenanthrenes are morphine, codeine, and thebaine, while the benzylisoquinolines do not have any known medicinal or recreational effect (DEA 2005).

Morphine

Morphine is the primary active ingredient of opium, where it ranges in concentration from 4% to 21%. Commercial opium is standardized to contain 10% morphine. In the United States, a small percentage of the morphine obtained from opium each year is used directly (about 20 tons); the remainder is converted into codeine and other derivatives (about 110 tons) (DEA 2005).

Morphine is one of the most effective drugs known for the relief of severe pain, and remains the standard against which new painkillers are measured. In the United States, oral morphine is the favored drug to treat severe pain associated with advanced-stage cancer (Pharo and Zhou 2005). As with most opioid painkillers, the use of morphine has increased significantly in the past decade. Since 1998, there has been about a two-fold increase in the use of morphine products in the United States (DEA 2005).

Morphine (full name morphine sulfate) is marketed under both generic and brand-name products that include MS-Contin, Oramorph SR, MSIR, Roxanol, Kadian, and RMS. Morphine is used by injection (parenterally) for preoperative sedation, as a supplement to surgical anesthesia, and for pain relief. Traditionally, morphine was almost exclusively used by injection. Today, morphine is sold in a variety of forms, including oral solutions, immediate- and sustained-release tablets and capsules, suppositories, and injectable preparations.

Codeine

Codeine was first isolated in 1832 and represents the earliest mild opioid-based painkiller (Trescot et al. 2008). The codeine alkaloid is found in opium in concentrations ranging from 0.7% to 2.5%, and codeine is the most widely used opioid derivative for medical use in the world. Most codeine used in the United States is produced from morphine, and codeine is also the precursor compound for the production of several semisynthetic opioids including hydrocodone. Codeine is used medically for the relief of moderate pain and cough suppression. Compared to morphine, codeine produces less analgesia, sedation, and respiratory depression (DEA 2005). Relative to morphine, codeine is approximately 60% as effective when taken orally versus by injection as an analgesic and respiratory depressant. Approximately 10% of ingested codeine is metabolized to morphine, and free and conjugated morphine is found in the urine after use of codeine. Codeine has a very low affinity for opioid receptors, and the analgesic effect of codeine is due to its conversion to morphine, not necessarily a direct effect of codeine itself. However, the antitussive (cough suppressing) effects of this drug may involve distinct receptors that bind codeine itself (Gutstein and Akil 2006).

Codeine is available in tablets either alone (schedule II) or in combination with aspirin or acetaminophen (that is, Tylenol with Codeine, schedule III). As a cough suppressant, codeine is found in a number of liquid preparations and cough syrups (schedule V). Codeine is also used to a lesser extent as an injectable solution for the treatment of pain. Codeine products are diverted from legitimate sources for nonmedical use (DEA 2005).

Codeine is susceptible to drug-drug interactions, especially by drugs that block its breakdown and inactivation such as bupropion (Wellbutrin), celecoxib (Celebrex), cimetidine, and cocaine, and drugs that speed up its breakdown and inactivation such as dexamethasone and rifampin (Trescot et al. 2008). Low doses of codeine can cause greater nausea and vomiting than high doses, an unexpected effect (Trescot et al. 2008).

Thebaine

Thebaine is a minor ingredient of opium. It is placed in the DEA schedule II and is also tightly regulated under international law. Although chemically similar to both morphine and codeine, thebaine produces a stimulant rather than a sedating effect. Thebaine is not used therapeutically, but instead is converted into a variety of substances such as oxycodone, oxymorphone, nalbuphine, naloxone, naltrexone, and buprenorphine. The United States ranks first in the world in the utilization of thebaine (DEA 2005).

Semisynthetic Opioid Agonists

The following opioids are among the more significant substances derived from the morphine, codeine, and thebaine contained in opium that have been in widespread medical use.

Heroin

Heroin (full chemical name diacetylmorphine hydrochloride) is produced by altering morphine. Heroin is generally believed to have no significant opioid receptor activity. Instead, once in the body heroin is rapidly metabolized to 6-monoacetylmorphine and then to morphine in the brain.

Diacetylmorphine and 6-monoacetylmorphine rapidly cross the blood-brain barrier, while morphine itself is much slower to do so; thus, the compound heroin is considered an inactive molecular appendage (or prodrug) to morphine that accelerates the entry of morphine into the brain (White and Irvine 1999).

Heroin is synthesized by collecting and converting powdered opium to heroin hydrochloride (Schwartz 1998).

Heroin rapidly enters the brain after injection, where it binds to mu, kappa, and other opiate-receptor binding sites (Schwartz 1998). Euphoria occurs approximately thirty minutes after nasal ingestion, fifteen minutes after intramuscular injection, and within a few seconds after intravenous injection. Heroin produces an effect that lasts about three to four hours (Schwartz 1998). As with many other opioids, heroin reduces the anticipatory anxiety associated with emotional or physical pain and alters the perception of pain (Schwartz 1998).

Other drugs such as tricyclic antidepressants can block and delay the metabolism of heroin (White and Irvine 1999).

Hydromorphone

Hydromorphone is derived from morphine and shares the pharmacologic properties of morphine and other mu-opioid agonists but is shorter acting and produces more sedation. Hydromorphone is 5 times as potent orally and 8.5 times as potent by injection than morphine, and can be administered by injection, by infusion, orally, and rectally (Sarhill, Walsh, and Nelson 2001).

Following oral ingestion of conventional-release hydromorphone, the drug is rapidly absorbed and undergoes hepatic first-pass elimination of approximately 50%. This means that half the drug is eliminated by the liver before it reaches the brain. The side effects are comparable to those of morphine (Sarhill, Walsh, and Nelson 2001).

Hydromorphone (Dilaudid) is marketed in tablets (2, 4, and 8 mg), suppositories, oral solutions, and injectable formulations. In September 2004, the FDA approved the extended-release formulation of hydromorphone hydrochloride for marketing as Palladone for the management of persistent severe pain. However, at the request of the FDA, this drug was withdrawn from the U.S. market the following July by its manufacturer, Purdue Pharma, over concerns related to toxicity when ingested with alcohol (FDA 2005). All hydromorphone products are DEA schedule II (DEA 2005). Hydromorphone is highly sought after by opioid addicts and is usually obtained through fraudulent prescriptions or theft. Hydromorphone tablets are often dissolved and injected as a substitute for heroin (DEA 2005).

Oxymorphone

Oxymorphone is derived from morphine and has a high affinity for the mu-opioid receptor and negligible interaction with kappa and delta opioid receptors (Prommer 2006). Oxymorphone, about ten times more potent than morphine, first received FDA approval for sale in the United States for pain relief in 1959. It has recently become available in immediate-release and sustained-release formulations (Opana, Numorphan, Numorphone) (Trescot et al. 2008).

Oxymorphone is an effective opioid analgesic with a safety profile comparable to that of other opioid drugs, though oxymorphone may be safer for elderly or frail patients who are also taking drugs that are metabolized by the same liver enzymes (Pergolizzi, Raffa, and Gould 2009).

Hydrocodone

Hydrocodone is a semisynthetic codeine derivative that closely resembles morphine in its pharmacological profile. Hydrocodone was first used medically as a cough suppressant and analgesic in the 1920s (Homsi, Walsh, and Nelson 2001; DEA 2005). Some of the metabolites (breakdown products) of hydrocodone are more powerful than hydrocodone itself. Thus, similar to codeine, it has been proposed that hydrocodone is a prodrug. Its analgesic properties are generally considered similar in potency to those of codeine (Otton et al. 1993; Cone et al. 2006).

As a drug of abuse, hydrocodone is similar to morphine in its subjective effects, opioid signs and symptoms, and "drug-liking" scores. Hydrocodone products are frequently abused and are the most frequently prescribed pharmaceutical opioids in the United States, with over 111 million prescriptions dispensed in 2003. In fact, more than 99% of the world's hydrocodone supply is used in the United States (Manchikanti 2007). Hydrocodone products are among the most popular prescription drugs associated with drug diversion, trafficking, abuse, and addiction. In every area in the country, the DEA has listed this drug as one of the most commonly diverted. Hydrocodone is the most frequently encountered opioid pharmaceutical in submissions of drug evidence to federal, state, and local forensic laboratories. Law enforcement has documented the diversion of millions of dosage units of hydrocodone by theft, doctor shopping, fraudulent prescriptions, bogus "call-in" prescriptions, and diversion by registrants and Internet fraud (DEA 2005). Poison control data, DAWN medical examiner (ME) data, and other ME data indicate that hydrocodone deaths are numerous, widespread, and increasing. In addition, the hydrocodone-acetaminophen combinations (accounting for about 80% of all hydrocodone prescriptions) pose significant health risks when taken in excess because of the harmful effect on the liver of excessive acetaminophen (DEA 2005).

Hydrocodone is an effective cough suppressant and analgesic. It is most frequently prescribed in combination with acetaminophen (Vicodin, Lortab) but is also marketed in products with aspirin (Lortab ASA), ibuprofen (Vicoprofen), and antihistamines (Hycomine). All products currently marketed in the United States are either schedule III combination products primarily intended for pain management or schedule V cough medications usually sold in liquid formulations. The schedule III products are currently under review at the federal level to determine if an increase in regulatory control is needed (DEA 2005). Schedule III medications have less regulatory control than schedule II medications, allowing for easier access and wider use. This contributes to the excessive prescribing and abuse of hydrocodone in the United States.

Oxycodone

Oxycodone is synthesized from thebaine and, like morphine and hydromorphone, is used medically as a pain reliever. Oxycodone is similar in structure to hydrocodone. Oxycodone is a pure mu-opioid receptor agonist that has been in medical use since 1917. Unlike codeine and hydrocodone, oxycodone is a potent analgesic in its own right and not a prodrug, although enzyme activity in the liver converts oxycodone into the active opioid analgesic metabolite oxymorphone (see prior section) during the process of breakdown and elimination. Oxycodone is primarily prescribed for oral use and may also be given IM, IV, subcutaneously, and rectally. In analgesic potency, oxycodone is comparable to morphine, and both drugs possess a similar abuse potential. With the exception of hallucinations, which occur more rarely with oxycodone than with morphine, the side effects of these drugs are very similar (Poyhia et al. 1992). Due to the breakdown products of oxycodone that are produced during metabolism, urine toxicology screens may reveal oxycodone alone, oxycodone and oxymorphone, or oxymorphone alone following the use of oxycodone (Leow et al. 1992).

The use of oxycodone has increased dramatically in the United States. In 2003, about 41 tons of oxycodone were manufactured for sale in the United States, compared with roughly 3.5 tons in 1993 (DEA 2005). Historically, oxycodone products have been popular drugs of abuse among the opiate-abusing population. In recent years, concern has grown among federal, state, and local officials over the huge increase in the illicit availability and abuse of OxyContin products which, unlike older formulations of oxycodone with 5 mg of drug, contain much larger amounts of oxycodone (10 to 80 mg) in a formulation intended for delayed release over a twelve-hour period. Abusers of oxycodone learned to circumvent the slow-release mechanism by crushing the tablet and swallowing, snorting, injecting, or smoking the drug. This drug alteration produces a dramatically more rapid and intense high. Addiction, fatal overdose, and the criminal activities associated with obtaining and distributing this drug have reached epidemic proportions in some areas of the United States (DEA 2005).

Oxycodone is marketed alone in 10, 20, 40, and 80 mg controlled-release tablets (OxyContin) and 5 mg immediate-release capsules (OxyIR). However, most oxycodone formulations also contain additional active ingredients such as acetaminophen, ibuprofen, homatropine methylbromide, chlorpheniramine maleate, phenylephrine, guaifenesin, and caffeine. Oxycodone in an immediate-release formulation is sold as Percocet and Percodan. Percocet comes in 2.5 mg, 5 mg, 7.5 mg, and 10 mg tablets. Percodan is a combination of oxycodone 4.8 mg with aspirin. All oxycodone products are DEA schedule II (DEA 2005). Distribution of the 160 mg dose of OxyContin was discontinued by Purdue Pharma in 2001 over concerns of abuse and diversion (USGAO 2003). The antidepressant drugs fluoxetine (Prozac) and sertraline (Zoloft) compete with oxycodone for the same liver enzyme for metabolism and clearance, and can potentially cause increased and prolonged elevations of oxycodone levels and toxicity (Davis et al. 2003).

Synthetic Opioid Agonists

In contrast to the pharmaceutical products described above that are derived from opium, synthetic narcotics are produced entirely within the laboratory. The continuing search for products that retain the analgesic properties of morphine without the risk of tolerance and dependence has yet to yield a product that is not susceptible to abuse. A number of clandestinely produced drugs, as well as drugs that have accepted medical uses, fall within this category (DEA 2005).

Meperidine

Introduced as an analgesic in the 1930s, meperidine's effects are similar, but not identical, to morphine's, with a shorter duration of action and less antitussive and antidiarrheal actions. Meperidine, predominantly a mu receptor agonist, is used for pre anesthesia and relief of moderate to severe pain, particularly in obstetrics and postoperative care. It is no longer recommended for the treatment of chronic pain because of concerns over metabolic toxicity and should not be used for longer than forty-eight hours. In equivalent pain-relieving doses, meperidine produces sedation, respiratory depression, and euphoria comparable to morphine, although some patients may experience dysphoria. Meperidine can produce a state of CNS excitation, characterized by tremors, muscle twitches, and in high doses, seizures that are primarily due to accumulation of the metabolite normeperidine. Also, large doses repeated at short intervals by addicts who have developed a tolerance to the sedative effects can produce an excitatory syndrome characterized by hallucinations, tremors, muscle twitches, dilated pupils, hyperactive reflexes, and convulsions (Gutstein and Akil 2006).

Meperidine is available in tablets, syrups, and injectable forms under generic and brand name (such as Demerol and Mepergan) schedule II preparations. Several analogues of meperidine have been clandestinely produced. During the clandestine synthesis of the analogue MPPP, a neurotoxic by-product (MPTP) was inadvertently produced. A number of individuals who consumed the MPPP/MPTP preparation developed an irreversible Parkinsonian-like syndrome. It was later found that MPTP destroys the same neurons as those damaged in Parkinson's disease (DEA 2005).

Methadone

Methadone was synthesized in Germany during World War II as an analgesic after their supply of raw opium from which to synthesize morphine was cut off (Krantz and Mehler 2004). Although chemically unlike morphine or heroin, methadone produces many of the same effects. It was introduced in the United States in 1947 as an analgesic (Dolophine). High-dose methadone can block the effects of heroin and other opioid drugs, thereby discouraging addicts from continuing opioid use, and it is the treatment of opioid addiction that has constituted the primary use of methadone in the United States over the last four decades. However, methadone is increasingly being used in the management of chronic pain. As with any opioid, chronic use of methadone leads to tolerance and dependence (DEA 2005).

Methadone is a long-acting mu receptor agonist with pharmacological properties similar to those of morphine (Gutstein and Akil 2006), and methadone's effects can last up to twenty-four hours, permitting once-a-day oral administration in heroin and other opioid detoxification and methadone maintenance programs (DEA 2005). Some of the outstanding properties of methadone are its analgesic activity, its effectiveness when taken orally, its extended duration of action in suppressing withdrawal symptoms in physically dependent opioid users, and its ability to demonstrate persistent effects with repeated administration (Gutstein and Akil 2006). One of the most important advantages of methadone is that it alleviates cravings for opioids—a primary reason for relapse—and blocks many of the pleasurable effects of heroin and other abused opioids, which helps to reinforce abstinence (Krantz and Mehler 2004). Methadone maintenance is the primary method of heroin addiction treatment in the United States. The more frequent side effects include sweating, decreased libido, weight gain, constipation, and irregular menstrual periods, occurring primarily during the initial stabilization process of long-term methadone treatment of opioid addiction (Krantz and Mehler 2004). Tolerance to the opioid effects of methadone develops within four weeks. The minimal effective dose in methadone maintenance is considered to be 50 mg, but some patients require much higher doses (Krantz and Mehler 2004), commonly in the range of 100–200 mg per day.

Following absorption, methadone is distributed to the brain, liver, kidneys, muscles, and lungs. Tissue binding predominates over binding to plasma proteins, and methadone accumulates in these tissues with repeated dosing. This binding of the drug to tissues and organs with repeated dosing creates a reservoir of methadone, which results in blood plasma concentrations being maintained. Methadone reabsorption from the reservoir tissues may continue for weeks after administration has ended (Garrido and Troconiz 1999). The long elimination half-life of about twenty-two hours, and the buildup of methadone in various tissue regions of the body, causes the withdrawal syndrome to develop more slowly upon cessation of use and to be less severe but more prolonged than that of heroin (DEA 2005).

In contrast to heroin, the activity of methadone is due almost exclusively to the parent drug rather than its metabolites. One of the primary elimination pathways of methadone involves the liver enzyme cytochrome P450 3A4. Medications that block the action of P450 3A4, such as ketoconazole and erythromycin, may enhance and prolong the effect of methadone; drugs that activate the P450 3A4 enzyme, such as rifampin, carbamazepine, and phenytoin, will have the opposite effect (White and Irvine 1999). Cocaine accelerates the elimination of methadone (Moolchan, Umbricht, and Epstein 2001). Several antiretroviral drugs used in the treatment of HIV infection interact with methadone to result in a decrease in methadone levels, and in some cases a methadone withdrawal syndrome. These drugs include abacavir (Ziagen) (Gourevitch 2001); lopinavir and ritonavir (Kaletra) (Chrisman 2003; McCance-Katz et al. 2002); nelfinavir (Viracept)

(McCance-Katz et al. 2004; Eap, Buclin, and Baumann 2002); and nevirapine (Viramune) (Eap, Buclin, and Baumann 2002; Gerber 2002). Increases in methadone dosing are necessary to counteract this effect with many of these drugs (Trescot et al. 2008). Heroin addicts have a high rate of HIV infection; thus knowledge of these drug interactions is essential to the treatment of those with both HIV infection and heroin addiction.

Subcutaneous administration of 10 to 20 mg methadone to opioid addicts in recovery unambiguously produces euphoria similar in duration and intensity to that of morphine, and its overall abuse potential is comparable with that of morphine (Gutstein and Akil 2006). Methadone is available in oral solutions, tablets, and injectable schedule II formulations (DEA 2005).

The four to eight hours of pain relief from methadone is much shorter than the elimination half-life of the drug, which can vary from 12 to 150 hours. This difference, plus the potential interaction with several other drugs, raises the risk of fatal toxicity when methadone is prescribed by an inexperienced or untrained physician, or when dosing for pain relief or euphoria is self-directed by the patient (Trescot et al. 2008).

LAAM

Closely related to methadone, the synthetic compound levo-alpha acetyl methadol, or LAAM (Orlaam), has an even longer duration of action (forty-eight to seventy-two hours) than methadone. LAAM was first developed by German chemists in 1948, and like methadone, LAAM has a high abuse potential (DEA 2005).

LAAM is a synthetic mu-opioid receptor agonist that is rapidly absorbed following oral administration. The clinical use of LAAM is based primarily on the activity of two metabolites, nor-LAAM and dinor-LAAM, and it is the combined activity of all three compounds that gives LAAM its long duration of action (Finn and Wilcock 1997). As early as 1952, LAAM was identified as an agent that could prevent opioid withdrawal symptoms for more than seventy-two hours. In 1993, the FDA approved LAAM for the treatment of opioid addiction (Finn and Wilcock 1997), and the use of LAAM in this context was intended to build on the strengths and improve on the drawbacks of methadone (Krantz and Mehler 2004). Similar to methadone, LAAM blocks the euphoric effects of other opioids while controlling opioid craving by producing a cross-tolerance to illicit opioid use. The ninety-minute onset of action is slower than methadone, but the duration of action is significantly longer, allowing dosing of three times per week. The average daily dose is 75 to 115 mg, and the side effects of LAAM are infrequent and are comparable to those of methadone (Krantz and Mehler 2004). However, concerns over cardiovascular toxicity and subsequent under-utilization led the manufacturer of LAAM to withdraw the drug from the U.S. market in 2004 (Krantz and Mehler 2004).

Propoxyphene

A close relative of methadone, propoxyphene was first marketed in 1957 under the trade name Darvon. Propoxyphene binds primarily to mu-opioid receptors to produce mild analgesic and other CNS effects similar to those seen with other mu receptor agonist opioids. Its painkilling potency is one-half to one-third that of codeine, with 65 mg roughly equivalent to about 600 mg of aspirin. The average half-life of propoxyphene in plasma after a single dose is longer than for codeine, six to twelve hours. Unpleasant side effects and the possibility of toxic psychoses make high-dose use of propoxyphene prohibitive, and very large doses produce respiratory depression in morphine-tolerant addicts, suggesting incomplete cross-tolerance between propoxyphene and morphine. Abuse via the IM or IV routes results in severe damage to veins and soft tissues (Gutstein and Akil 2006). Individuals who are lacking the key liver enzyme that converts hydrocodone into its active form report superior pain relief from propoxyphene because a different group of liver enzymes are involved in its breakdown (Trescot et al. 2008).

More than 150 tons of propoxyphene are produced every year in the United States, with more than 25 million prescriptions written for propoxyphene products. The toxic side effects of this drug contribute to making it among the top ten drugs reported by medical examiners in drug abuse deaths (DEA 2005). The widespread popularity of propoxyphene as a drug of abuse is largely a result of unfounded concern about the addictive potential of codeine by prescribing physicians (Gutstein and Akil 2006).

Propoxyphene is prescribed for relief of mild to moderate pain. Preparations containing it, such as Darvon and Darvocet, are schedule IV medications (DEA 2005).

The *New York Times* reported on January 31, 2009, that medical advisors to the FDA recommended the removal of this drug from the market by a vote of fourteen to twelve. This vote was the response to the request of a watchdog group, Public Citizen, that the drug be pulled from the market due to inadequate pain relief properties and significant overdose risk *(New York Times* 2009).

Fentanyl

First synthesized in Belgium in the late 1950s, fentanyl has an analgesic potency about eighty times that of morphine. It was introduced into U.S. medical practice in the 1960s as an intravenous anesthetic under the trade name Sublimaze. Two other fentanyl analogues were subsequently introduced: alfentanil (Alfenta), an ultra-short (five to ten minutes) acting analgesic, and sufentanil (Sufenta), an exceptionally potent analgesic (one thousand times more potent than morphine) for use in heart surgery. The fentanyls are extensively used for anesthesia and analgesia. Duragesic is a fentanyl transdermal patch used in chronic pain management, and Actiq is a solid formulation of fentanyl citrate on a stick, resembling a lollipop, that dissolves slowly in the mouth for transmucosal absorption. Actiq is intended for opioid-tolerant individuals and is effective in treating breakthrough pain in cancer patients. Carfentanil citrate (Wildnil) is an analogue of fentanyl with an analgesic potency ten thousand times that of morphine and is used in veterinary practice to immobilize large animals (DEA 2005).

Fentanyl is a synthetic opioid related to the phenylpiperidine class of opioid molecules, and the actions of fentanyl and its congeners—sufentanil, remifentanil, and alfentanil—are similar to those of the other mu receptor agonists. However, the fentanyls are distinguished from other opioids by their shorter time to peak analgesic effect, rapid termination of effect after small doses, and relative cardiovascular stability, which has made their use during surgery very popular. The time to peak analgesia is rapid, approximately five minutes. The respiratory depression potential is similar to other mu receptor agonists, with a more rapid onset. Fentanyl and sufentanil treatment of chronic pain, particularly in the formulation of Duragesic, has become much more prevalent in the past decade (Gutstein and Akil 2006).

The nonmedical use and abuse of pharmaceutical fentanyl was first observed in the mid-1970s in the medical community and continues to be a problem in the United States and worldwide. Anesthesia personnel are the most likely to abuse these medications, because they have the most access to them. Due to their high potency, these are extremely dangerous medications to abuse and are highly likely to cause death by respiratory depression. To date, more than twelve different analogues of fentanyl have been produced clandestinely and identified in the U.S. drug traffic. The biological effects of the fentanyls are indistinguishable from those of heroin, though fentanyls can be hundreds of times more potent. Fentanyls are most commonly used by IV administration, but like heroin, they may also be smoked or snorted (DEA 2005).

Fentanyl comes in a transdermal formulation, or patch, that is delivered via the skin for up to seventy-two hours, with the patches containing 2.5, 5, 7.5, or 10 mg of fentanyl. As with the injectable formulation of fetanyl (Sublimaze), Duragesic abuse is primarily, but not exclusively, a problem with health care professionals because of their access to supplies of the drug. Abusers extract the fetanyl from the patch to inject, chew, ingest, or inhale the patch contents (Ling, Wesson, and Smith 2005).

Tramadol

Tramadol (Ultram) is a synthetic codeine analogue that does not fit into any of the standard classes of opioid drugs. A unique painkiller, tramadol is a partial mu agonist and has activity with other brain chemicals that include GABA, norepinephrine, and serotonin (Trescot et al. 2008), all of which contribute to its painkilling properties (Gutstein and Akil 2006). Tramadol is as effective as morphine or meperidine in the treatment of mild to moderate pain. The affinity of tramadol for the mu-opioid receptor is only 1/6,000 that of morphine, although the primary metabolite of tramadol is two to four times as potent as the parent drug and may partially explain the analgesic effect. Physical dependence with tramadol has been reported (Gutstein and Akil 2006) and addiction noted among medical personnel and others. A study that included interviews with large numbers of chronic pain patients found the abuse potential of tramadol comparable to that of NSAIDS (nonsteroidal anti-inflammatory drugs) (Adams et al. 2006). Tramadol addiction is regularly seen among health care professionals in addiction treatment programs. Tramadol is currently not a controlled substance by the DEA, and although it is used primarily as an analgesic, it has demonstrated usefulness in treating opioid withdrawal (Threlkeld et al. 2006; Trescot et al. 2008).

Levorphanol

Levorphanol (Levo-Dromoran) is the only commercially available opioid agonist of the morphinan series and possesses pharmacological effects very similar to those of morphine. It was first synthesized more than forty years ago as a pharmacological alternative to morphine and has a greater potency than morphine. The analgesia produced by levorphanol is mediated by its interactions with the mu, delta, and kappa opioid receptors. Levorphanol also blocks the activity of the NMDA receptor (Prommer 2007), which may account for its effectiveness in treating pain of neuropathic origin (Trescot et al. 2008).

The long half-life of the drug, twelve to sixteen hours, increases the potential for drug accumulation. Levorphanol has clinical efficacy in neuropathic pain (Prommer 2007) and recently interest has increased in using levorphanol for the treatment of refractory pain (Trescot et al. 2008).

Diphenoxylate and Loperamide

Diphenoxylate (Lomotil) and loperamide (Imodium) are meperidine congeners that are FDA-approved for the treatment of diarrhea. Both drugs slow gastrointestinal movement through affecting the circular and longitudinal muscles of the intestine, presumably by interacting with opioid receptors in the intestine (Gutstein and Akil 2006).

Lomotil comes in tablet and liquid, and each tablet and each 5 ml liquid contains diphenoxylate hydrochloride 2.5 mg and atropine sulfate 0.025 mg. The atropine is included in the formulation to discourage nonmedical use and abuse. The following atropine sulfate effects are listed in decreasing order of severity, but not of frequency: hyperthermia, tachycardia, urinary retention, flushing, dryness of the skin and mucous membranes (package insert, G.D. Searle 2006). Overuse is readily discouraged by these side effects.

Diphenoxylate has essentially no morphine-like subjective effects at therapeutic doses, but at high doses produces codeine-like effects. The dose that produces antidiarrheal action is considerably lower than the dose that causes central nervous system effects. It is very difficult to turn diphenoxylate into a liquid solution, which prevents intravenous use. A dose of 100 to 300 mg/day, which is equivalent to 40 to 120 tablets, administered to humans for 40 to 70 days, produced opioid withdrawal symptoms and suggests that addiction to diphenoxylate is possible at high doses. Lomotil is classified as a DEA schedule V controlled substance (package insert, G.D. Searle 2006).

Loperamide produces little effect on the central nervous system due to difficulty in crossing the blood-brain barrier for entry into the brain, and it is this lack of effect on the brain that gives the drug little if any abuse potential (Baker 2007). Despite the perceived lack of abuse liability (Jaffe, Kanzler, and Green 1980), several reports of loperamide abuse have been documented (Langlitz, Schotte, and Bschor 2001; Katz and Sturmann 1993).

Each capsule of Imodium contains loperamide hydrochloride 2 mg. Tiredness, dizziness, or drowsiness may occur during initial therapy with loperamide. Loperamide has not been placed on the DEA controlled substance schedule and is available over the counter (Loperamide package insert, Teva Pharmaceuticals USA 2006).

Mixed Agonist/Antagonists

Discovery of an opioid analgesic with the effectiveness but not the side effects or abuse potential of mu-opioid agonists such as morphine has been the Holy Grail of analgesic research for the past fifty years (Woolf and Hashmi 2004). Mixed agonist-antagonist compounds were developed with the hope that they would have less addictive potential and create less respiratory depression than morphine and related drugs. However, achieving the same degree of pain relief with these drugs produces a similar magnitude of side effects, and a ceiling effect occurs, both of which limit the potential pain relief. Also, some mixed agonist-antagonist drugs, such as pentazocine and nalorphine, can produce side effects not often seen with pure agonists, such as severe psychoses, that are not reversible with the opiate antagonist naloxone (Trescot et al. 2008; Gutstein and Akil 2006).

Drugs such as nalbuphine and butorphanol are mu receptor antagonists, and their painkilling properties are due to action as a kappa receptor agonist. Pentazocine qualitatively resembles these drugs, but is a weaker mu receptor antagonist or partial agonist while retaining its kappa agonist activity (Gutstein and Akil 2006).

Pentazocine

The effort to find an effective analgesic with a lower potential for abuse and dependence than morphine led to the development of pentazocine (Talwin), which was introduced to the U.S. market as an analgesic in 1967 (DEA 2005). With both agonist and weak antagonistic activity, the pattern of central nervous system effects with pentazocine is similar to that of morphine-like opioids, including analgesia, sedation, and respiratory depression. Dysphoria and psychosis can be precipitated by higher doses in the range of 60 to 90 mg (Gutstein and Akil 2006).

Following its introduction to the U.S. market, pentazocine was frequently encountered in the illicit market, usually in combination with the antihistamine tripelennamine, and was placed in DEA schedule IV in 1979. Reducing the abuse of this drug was accomplished with the introduction of Talwin Nx. This product contains a quantity of naloxone, an opioid receptor antagonist, sufficient to counteract the morphine-like effects of pentazocine if the tablets are dissolved and injected (DEA 2005). When taken orally, naloxone passes through the body and is eliminated without being activated.

Nalbuphine

Nalbuphine (Nubain) is a mixed opioid agonist-antagonist related to naloxone and oxymorphone. It has a spectrum of effects that qualitatively resembles that of pentazocine but with a lower likelihood of producing dysphoric side effects. Although doses of 10 mg or less produce few side effects, much higher doses (more than 70 mg) can produce psychological side effects such as dysphoria, racing thoughts, and distorted body image. Prolonged administration of nalbuphine can produce physical dependence, and the withdrawal syndrome is similar in intensity to that seen with pentazocine (Gutstein and Akil 2006).

Butorphanol

While butorphanol can be made from the opium constituent thebaine, it is typically manufactured synthetically. Butorphanol acts similar to pentazocine and is more suitable for the relief of acute pain than chronic pain. The primary side effects include drowsiness, weakness, sweating, feelings of floating, and nausea. Although the incidence of psychotic-like side effects is lower than with comparable doses of pentazocine, they are similar in quality. Physical dependence on butorphanol can develop from regular use (Gutstein and Akil 2006).

Butorphanol was initially available in injectable forms for human (Stadol) and veterinary (Torbugesic and Torbutrol) use. A nasal spray (Stadol NS) resulted in significant diversion and abuse of this product, which led to its 1997 assignment as a DEA schedule IV substance. Butorphanol is an example of a drug gaining favor as a drug of abuse after its introduction in a formulation that facilitated greater ease of administration (nasal spray versus injection) (DEA 2005).

Partial Agonists

Buprenorphine

Buprenorphine is a semisynthetic opioid first derived from thebaine in 1966. It was first suggested in 1978 as an alternative to methadone for opioid replacement therapy with heroin addicts (Davids and Gastpar 2004). In December 1981, this drug was approved by the FDA for use in pain relief in the United States (Trescot et al. 2008). France was the first country to use buprenorphine to treat opioid addiction, in 1996 (Reisinger 2006). The Drug Addiction Treatment Act of 2000 allowed for qualified physicians to prescribe it for maintenance treatment of opioid addiction in the United States. The brands Suboxone and Subutex were made available for this use in January 2003.

Buprenorphine has a very low oral bioavailability (rate of absorption) because of substantial intestinal and hepatic metabolism before entry into the bloodstream. The sublingual (under the tongue) formulation used to treat opioid addiction is adequately absorbed, and maximum blood plasma level is achieved seventy to ninety minutes following sublingual administration. Following absorption, buprenorphine initially accumulates in organs such as the liver, kidneys, muscular tissue, and finally fatty tissue, where it is released when the blood plasma level drops (Davids and Gastpar 2004). This is very similar to methadone—a reservoir-like situation allows for an extended period of drug availability as it leaks out of these tissues. The minimum daily dose needed to suppress opioid abuse is about 4 mg. Doses usually do not exceed 32 mg, as little therapeutic benefit occurs above that level (Davids and Gastpar 2004). Buprenorphine may trigger withdrawal in patients who have received repeated doses of a morphine-like opioid agonist and have developed physical dependence. It must be used carefully to avoid such a reaction. However, it does not produce the psychotic-like effects seen with the mixed agonist-antagonists (Inturrisi 2002).

Buprenorphine should not be used with alcohol; cases of lethal intoxication with buprenorphine almost always involve abuse of another substance such as alcohol or sedatives (Davids and Gastpar 2004). Upon discontinuation, a withdrawal syndrome develops from two days to two weeks later, with signs and symptoms typical of a milder morphine-type withdrawal lasting roughly one to two weeks (Gutstein and Akil 2006). The more benign withdrawal syndrome is due to the partial agonist property at the mu receptor and weak antagonist property at the kappa receptor of buprenorphine (Krantz and Mehler 2004). However, clinical descriptions of significant withdrawal symptoms, not unlike those from methadone, are commonplace. This usually involves anxiety, sleeplessness, and low energy. Craving is very high during this period.

Buprenorphine was initially marketed in the United States as an analgesic (Buprenex). In 2002, two new products (Suboxone and Subutex) were oproved for the treatment of opiate addiction. Similar to methadone and ΛM, buprenorphine is very potent (thirty to fifty times the analgesic cy of morphine), has a long duration of action, and does not need to be injected to achieve therapeutic effectiveness. Unlike the other two drugs used in the treatment of opioid addiction, buprenorphine produces far less respiratory depression and is thought to be safer in overdose due to the "ceiling effect" that limits therapeutic effects at a certain level. All buprenorphine products are DEA schedule III (DEA 2005).

The Suboxone formulation of buprenorphine contains naloxone, which has little to no oral or sublingual absorption. Its purpose in the formulation is to deter IV or IM administration by those seeking to abuse the drug, since naloxone is an opioid antagonist that becomes active with IV or IM administration and blocks the desired opioid effect of the buprenorphine. The naloxone contained in Suboxone will also trigger sudden, severe opioid withdrawal in patients with ongoing opioid use (Trescot et al. 2008).

Physiological and Behavioral Effects of Prescription Opiates

Morphine and most other opioid agonists share the following physiological effects: analgesia; changes in mood and reward behavior; and alteration of respiratory cardiovascular, gastrointestinal, and neuroendocrine function (Gutstein and Akil 2006). As the dose of an opioid drug is increased, the subjective, analgesic (pain relief), and toxic effects become more pronounced. Except in cases of acute intoxication, there is no loss of motor coordination or slurred speech such as that found with many other drugs that produce a calming or sedating effect (DEA 2005).

Immediate and Short-Term Effects

Analgesia (Pain Relief)

Morphine-like drugs produce analgesia, drowsiness, changes in mood, and mental clouding, all without a loss of consciousness. Patients in pain report that the pain is less intense, less discomforting, or entirely absent when given therapeutic doses of these drugs. The pain relief is fairly selective, with other sensory perceptions unaffected. Some patients experience euphoria depending on the dose. When morphine in the same dose is continued

Table 7.1

Prescription Opioids Available in the United States

Drug name	Trade name	Category	Year introduced	Mechanism of action	DEA schedule
Opium	Laudanum, Paregoric	Natural opiate	Used throughout history	Mu agonist	II
Morphine sulfate	MS-Contin, Oramorph SR, MSIR, Roxanol, Kadian, RMS	Natural opiate	1830	Mu agonist	II
Codeine	Tylenol with Codeine, others	Natural opiate	1832	Mu agonist	III–V when combined with OTC analgesics or as cough syrup
Thebaine	None, used as a precursor for other opiates	Natural opiate	Not used medicinally	Mu agonist	II
Diacetyl-morphine	Heroin	Semisynthetic	1898	Mu agonist	I; no longer legal as a medicine
Hydromorphone	Dilaudid, others	Semisynthetic	1926	Mu agonist	II
Hydrocodone	Vicodin, others	Semisynthetic	1923	Mu agonist	III for tablets; V for cough syrup

Table 7.1

Prescription Opioids Available in the United States (cont'd.)

Drug name	Trade name	Category	Year introduced	Mechanism of action	DEA schedule
Oxymorphone	Numorphan	Semisynthetic	1959	Mu agonist	II
Oxycodone	OxyContin, Percocet, others	Semisynthetic	1917	Mu agonist	II
Meperidine	Demerol, others	Synthetic	1935	Mu agonist	II
Methadone	Dolophine, others	Synthetic	1943	Mu agonist	II
Levo-alpha acetyl methadol	LAAM, Orlaam	Synthetic	1948	Mu agonist	II
Propoxyphene	Darvon, Darvocet	Synthetic	1957	Mu agonist	IV
Fentanyl	Sublimaze, Actiq	Synthetic	1965	Mu agonist	II
Tramadol	Ultram	Synthetic	1972	Mu agonist, serotonin and norephinephrine reuptake inhibitor	Not on DEA schedule
Levorphanol	Levo-Dromoran	Synthetic	1953	Mu agonist	II

continued

Table 7.1

Prescription Opioids Available in the United States (cont'd.)

Drug name	Trade name	Category	Year introduced	Mechanism of action	DEA schedule
Diphenoxylate, loperamide	Lomotil, Imodium	Synthetic	1960, 1976	Mu agonist	V, OTC
Pentazocine	Talwin	Synthetic	1967	Mixed agonist-antagonist	IV
Nalbuphine	Nubain	Synthetic	1979	Mixed agonist-antagonist	Not on DEA schedule
Butorphanol	Stadol	Synthetic	1978	Mixed agonist-antagonist	IV
Buprenorphine	Buprenex, Suboxone, Subutex	Synthetic	1978	Partial agonist	III

given to a pain-free individual who is not an active or recovering drug or alcohol addict, the experience may be unpleasant. Nausea is a common experience in individuals taking morphine-like drugs, and vomiting may occur as well as drowsiness, a sluggish thought process, apathy, and decreased physical activity. The subjective, analgesic, and toxic effects, including respiratory depression, become more pronounced as the dose is increased. Morphine-like drugs seldom cause slurred speech, emotional breakdowns, or significant motor incoordination (Gutstein and Akil 2006).

Effect on Mood and Reward

Although the mechanisms by which opioids induce euphoria, tranquility, and other alterations of mood (including rewarding properties) are not entirely understood, the brain systems responsible for producing the opioid reinforcement are distinct from those involved in the development of physical dependence and analgesia (Koob and Bloom 1988). Behavioral and pharmacological data point to the role of dopamine pathways, particularly involving the nucleus accumbens (NAcc), in drug-induced reward, with interactions between opioids and dopamine producing the opioid-induced reinforcement (Gutstein and Akil 2006). This can cause loss of libido in men and menstrual irregularities in women.

Endocrine Effects

Morphine and similar drugs act in the hypothalamus to inhibit the release of gonadotropin-releasing hormone and corticotropin-releasing hormone, which decrease circulating luteinizing hormone, follicle-stimulating hormone, adrenocorticotropic hormone (ACTH), and beta-endorphin, which in turn reduce the plasma concentration of testosterone and cortisol (Gutstein and Akil 2006).

Miosis (Pupil Constriction)

Morphine and other opioid agonists constrict the pupils by stimulating the parasympathetic nerve that innervates the pupil (Gutstein and Akil 2006). Pinpoint pupils are a classic sign of opioid use.

Respiration

Morphine-like opioids slow the rate of breathing in part through a direct effect on the brain-stem respiratory center. Studies have shown that therapeutic doses of morphine depress all phases of respiratory activity, including rate, minute volume, and tidal exchange, and by possibly inducing irregular and periodic breathing. It appears that all opioid agonists can cause respiratory depression. Clinically significant respiratory depression seldom occurs at standard therapeutic doses. The primary mechanism of respiratory depression involves a reduced sensitivity of the brain-stem respiratory center to carbon dioxide (Gutstein and Akil 2006). Respiratory depression is the primary cause of death in opioid overdose.

Cough

Morphine and related opioids depress the cough reflex in part through direct action on the cough center in the medulla (Gutstein and Akil 2006).

Nauseant and Emetic Effects

Morphine-like drugs directly stimulate the chemoreceptor trigger zone for vomiting in the brain, resulting in nausea and vomiting in some patients (Gutstein and Akil 2006).

Gastrointestinal Effects

Morphine decreases gastric movement; diminishes biliary, pancreatic, and intestinal secretions; and delays the digestion of food in the small intestine. In the large intestine, peristaltic waves (the normal muscle movement of the gut) are diminished or eliminated and tone is increased to the point of spasm, delaying the passage of bowel contents (Gutstein and Akil 2006).

Effects of Chronic Use

The short-term use of opioids is associated with some well-known side effects such as nausea, sedation, euphoria, constipation, and itching. However, with chronic use, different types of side effects can develop, including hormonal and immune system effects, abuse and addiction, tolerance, and hyperalgesia (increased sensation of pain). More important, chronic medicinal opioid use has been linked with increases in disability, medical costs, and subsequent surgery (Manchikanti and Singh 2008).

Among the hazards of illicit drug use is the escalating risk of infection, disease, and overdose. Medical complications common among opioid abusers arise primarily from the impurities found in street drugs and in the nonsterile practices of injecting. Skin, lung, and brain abscesses, endocarditis (inflammation and infection of the lining of the heart), hepatitis, and HIV are commonly found among opioid abusers who inject their drugs. The physical signs of opioid overdose include constricted (pinpoint) pupils, cold clammy skin, confusion, convulsions, severe drowsiness, and respiratory depression (slow or troubled breathing). Most opioid deaths are the result of respiratory depression, where the person's breathing progressively slows and finally stops altogether (DEA 2005).

With the repeated use of opioids, tolerance develops to the desired effects of the drug. Tolerance is characterized by a shortened duration and a decreased intensity of pain relief, euphoria, and sedation, which creates the need to consume progressively larger doses to recapture the desired effect. Tolerant users can consume doses that far exceed their initial dose, and which are large enough to be fatal to someone who has not developed tolerance (DEA 2005). Tolerance to euphoria develops at a different rate than tolerance to other effects like respiratory depression. This can result in overdose, as one uses higher doses to increase intoxicating effects, while taking enough to slow breathing. *Cross-tolerance* refers to the same degree of tolerance to opioid effects when another opioid drug is used in place of the original opioid.

In patients taking opioid drugs for analgesia, increasing the dose can continue to provide adequate pain relief, and there does not appear to be a ceiling effect, beyond which no further pain relief can be obtained. However, higher doses can increase undesired side effects, such as nausea, vomiting, constipation, abdominal pain, and itching, which may limit the use of the drug (Pharo and Zhou 2005).

Hyperalgesia

Although prescription opioids have been and will continue to be used for the treatment of chronic pain, there is increasing recognition of the problem of *hyperalgesia* in patients receiving long-term opioid therapy. Opioid-induced hyperalgesia (OIH) is the process by which long-term mu-opioid agonist use actually leads to the increase in the sensation of pain. It is a growing concern because of the large number of patients receiving chronic opioid therapy. OIH is similar but not identical to the development of tolerance. The development of OIH is not well understood, but people experience pain from stimuli that would not have caused the same level of pain prior to the use of opioids. It seems as though the original pain problem is worse, so opioids are increased, actually causing more pain. Stopping opioids relieves the pain. Hyperalgesia is accompanied by allodynia—a painful response to a non-painful stimulus. People experiencing allodynia may feel pain when a piece of clothing rubs across their skin, for example. They have become extremely sensitive to painful and non-painful stimuli (Silverman 2009). Often those with chronic pain and opioid addiction no longer experience pain after discontinuation of opioids. It's as if they have been relieved of pain by stopping the opioids.

Opioids are incredibly effective analgesic agents. We are gaining neuro-biological understanding of how they work and how pain is experienced. However, we still have much to learn, as demonstrated by the controversies regarding chronic pain and the unusual nature of hyperalgesia.

CHAPTER 8

The OxyContin Story

The story of OxyContin is fascinating and unique. Although the United States has experienced several waves of widespread abuse of prescription medications during the past 150 years, the phenomenal, rapid ascent of OxyContin from market entry to miracle drug for those in chronic pain to a demonized substance being abused and diverted on a vast scale is the result of the confluence of several factors.

Changing Attitudes toward Pain Treatment

The 1990s witnessed a profound shift in the approach taken by physicians who treated patients suffering from pain. For most of the twentieth century, the pervasive viewpoint of the medical field was that patients given prescription opioids had a high risk of developing an addiction to them. This erroneous view meant that people suffering from cancer and other ailments involving serious and chronic pain were denied drugs that could have alleviated their suffering. During the 1990s a very different viewpoint emerged that was championed both by doctors specializing in pain treatment and by drug companies eager to broaden the market for such drugs. This viewpoint held that these medications posed little risk to pain patients.

Some experts now believe that this swing in the opposite direction of the traditionally held view on the addictive potential of prescription opioids had the unfortunate consequence of providing physicians with a false sense of security about these drugs (Meier 2003). It has also revealed the usefulness of opioids in the treatment of acute pain, and their disappointing results in the treatment of chronic pain.

These views of the threat prescription opioids pose to patients were shaped in the mid-1980s when pain treatment experts reported that cancer patients taking opioids did not experience the type of euphoria displayed by people who abused these drugs. This led some physicians to argue that strong, long-acting opioids could also be used safely to treat patients with serious pain unrelated to cancer, such as chronic back pain. The "pain management movement" helped improve the treatment of those with pain. Experts in the field were citing studies that they said validated their argument that powerful prescription opiate drugs posed a minimal risk of addiction when used in pain treatment (Meier 2003).

Drug companies underscored this theme in the marketing materials they sent to doctors and pharmacists. An example is Janssen Pharmaceutica, the producer of the fentanyl transdermal patch Duragesic, which described the risk of addiction to its product as "relatively rare" in a package insert with the drug. Endo Pharmaceuticals termed the risk "very rare" in presentations to hospital pharmacists. Purdue Pharma, the manufacturer of OxyContin, distributed a brochure to chronic pain patients titled "From One Pain Patient to Another," suggesting that OxyContin and similar drugs posed minimal risks. This brochure stated, "Some patients may be afraid of taking opioids because they are perceived as too strong or addictive, but that is far from actual fact. Less than 1 percent of patients taking opioids actually become addicted" (Meier 2003). These claims are far from the truth.

Many medical professionals did not realize there had not been any studies investigating the experience of pain patients who used long-acting opioids for extended periods of time. This led prescription opioid advocates and drug companies like Purdue Pharma to utilize data taken out of context from surveys of patients whose use of opioids was limited. An often-cited survey of opioid use from 1980 found "only four cases of addiction among 11,882 hospitalized patients." The lead researcher of that survey, Dr. Hershel Jick, an associate professor of medicine at Boston University, stated that his study did not follow patients after they left the hospital and did not address the risk of opioid abuse when they were pre-scribed in outpatient settings (Meier 2003). Other studies frequently cited data from cancer pain and addiction, not the more common chronic pain syndromes associated with low back pain and arthritis.

In addition to the pain management movement, shifting demographics played a role in the changing attitudes toward prescribing opioid drugs. As the incidence of painful diseases grew along with the overall age of the population, there was a growing acknowledgment of the importance of providing effective pain relief (USGAO 2003). Also during this period, national and international medical organizations began to develop and publish guidelines for the treatment of pain, which had an additional influence on the prescribing practices involving opioid drugs. In 1986, the highly influential World Health Organization (WHO 1986) determined that cancer pain could be relieved in most if not all patients, and encouraged physicians to prescribe opioid painkillers. WHO developed a three-step analgesic "ladder" as a practice guideline—a sequential use of different drugs for cancer pain management. For the first pain step, treatment with non-opioid analgesics such as aspirin or ibuprofen was recommended. If pain was not relieved, then an opioid such as codeine should be used for mild to moderate pain as the second step. For the third step—moderate to severe pain—opioids such as morphine should be used (USGAO 2003).

In 1995, the American Pain Society recommended treating pain as the fifth vital sign (along with pulse, blood pressure, core temperature, and respiration) to ensure that it would become common practice for health care providers to ask about pain during patient evaluations. The practice guidelines issued by the Agency for Health Care Policy and Research provided physicians and other health care professionals with information on the management of acute pain in 1992 and cancer pain in 1994. Health care providers and hospitals were further required to ensure that their patients received appropriate pain treatment when the Joint Commission on Accreditation of Healthcare Organizations (JCAHO), a national health care facility standards-setting and accrediting body, implemented its pain standards for hospital accreditation in 2001 (USGAO 2003). Even the U.S. Congress became involved in the shift to more aggressive pain management by passing a law in 2000 declaring the next ten years the "Decade of Pain Control and Research" (Kalb 2001).

In this environment, pharmaceutical companies began researching and developing new formulations of painkillers, and existing painkillers themselves became more widely prescribed than ever before. While the pharmaceutical market doubled to $145 billion between 1996 and 2000, the painkiller market tripled to $1.8 billion over the same period. Yet at the same time, reports of first-time abuse of painkillers also surged (Kalb 2001).

Advances in Drug Technology in the 1990s

Until the 1990s, the use of schedule II prescription opioid painkillers was primarily limited to operating rooms and inpatient settings because they had to be administered intravenously or intramuscularly, posing a serious obstacle to patients who needed powerful opioids to control disabling pain conditions. In response to this limitation, several pharmaceutical products were introduced to the market. Many of these newer agents were high-dose, extended-release formulations of pre-existing opioids, which included OxyContin (a new formulation of oxycodone), MS-Contin (a new formulation of morphine sulfate), and Palladone XL (a new formulation of hydromorphone hydrochloride). Each of these drugs met a genuine need by providing an elevated, constant blood level of the painkiller for extended periods, without the fluctuations of the short-acting formulations of the same opioid. These long-acting formulations reduced both the euphoric effects of the drug and pain more effectively by suppressing pain before it became established (preemptive effect) rather than treating it after, when higher doses might be required (Woolf and Hashmi 2004). By suppressing pain in this manner, the treatment could prevent chronic pain syndromes. Also, the controlled-release feature of OxyContin allowed a tablet to contain much more of the active ingredient than other, non-controlled-release oxycodone-containing drugs (USGAO 2003).

Product Launch

Near the end of 1995, the FDA approved Purdue Pharma's new highly potent, long-acting opioid painkiller OxyContin for the treatment of moderate to severe pain (Aquina et al. 2009). To help ensure a successful product launch, Purdue employed several innovative strategies to elevate the visibility and encourage the prescribing of its product.

In addition to placing doctor-directed ads in professional journals such as the *Journal of the American Medical Association,* Purdue began a novel indirect-marketing campaign just before the launch of OxyContin. Due to FDA marketing regulations on opioid-based drugs, the company was unable to use direct-to-consumer advertising, so Purdue concentrated on what it referred to as "nonbranded education." Just as Nike advertises the concept of sports instead of shoes, Purdue marketed the concept of pain relief to consumers, but without explicitly mentioning OxyContin. In 1994, the company launched Partners Against Pain, a public education program that initially focused on cancer pain and later addressed other forms of chronic pain. Through videos, patient pain journals, and an elaborate website, Purdue promoted three key messages to doctors and patients: (1) that pain was much more widespread than had previously been thought; (2) that pain was treatable; and (3) that in many cases pain could, and should, be treated with opioids. Purdue predicted that even without promoting OxyContin, Partners Against Pain would expand the total market, thereby increasing the number of prescriptions for OxyContin, and with it, the company's bottom line (Tough 2001).

The Explosive Growth in OxyContin Sales

Following its approval by the FDA, OxyContin was hailed as a breakthrough drug in the treatment of moderate to severe pain, and was viewed by many as a "miracle drug" because it allowed patients with chronic pain to achieve pain relief and resume a normal life (U.S. Department of Health and Human Services 2001). During the next few years, sales of OxyContin exploded. In a little more than four years, OxyContin's sales hit $1 billion, more than even that of Viagra (Meier and Peterson 2001). The revenue generated by OxyContin prescriptions for Purdue jumped from $44.8 million in 1996 to $981.6 million in 2000, $1.35 billion in 2001, and $1.53 billion in 2002. In 2000, doctors in the United States wrote almost 6 million OxyContin prescriptions (USGAO 2003). In 2001 and 2002 combined, sales of OxyContin approached $3 billion, more than 14 million prescriptions were dispensed, and OxyContin became the top-selling opioid, ranked as the fifteenth best-selling prescription drug in the country (as measured by retail sales) (USGAO 2003), and accounted for close to 80% of revenue for Purdue Pharma (Inciardi and Goode 2003). Fortuitous timing may have contributed to this phenomenal growth in sales of OxyContin, as the drug was launched during the national focus on the inadequacy of pain management (USGAO 2003). Table 8.1 summarizes the rapid increase in prescriptions and revenues of OxyContin from 1996 to 2002.

Table 8.1

OxyContin Sales and Prescriptions, 1996–2002

Year	Sales	Increase from previous year	Number of prescriptions	Increase from previous year
1996	$44,790,000	N/A	316,786	N/A
1997	$125,464,000	180%	924,375	192%
1998	$286,486,000	128%	1,910,944	107%
1999	$555,239,000	94%	3,504,827	83%
2000	$981,643,000	77%	5,932,981	69%
2001	$1,354,717,000	38%	7,183,327	21%
2002	$1,536,816,000	13%	7,234,204	7%

USGAO 2003

Purdue also attempted to expand the prescription opioid market beyond cancer patients, and its aggressive promotion of OxyContin for noncancer pain was an extraordinary success. In 1996, cancer patients were the primary market for long-acting opioids, but by 2000, only 3% of prescriptions written for OxyContin were made by oncologists. The treatment of pain with opioids was primarily done by pain experts, not primary care physicians. According to data by IMS Health, an information service providing pharmaceutical market research, the annual number of noncancer prescriptions for OxyContin increased nearly 1,000%, from about 670,000 in 1997 to roughly 6.2 million in 2002, whereas the annual number of OxyContin prescriptions for cancer-associated pain grew fourfold in six years from 250,000 to just over 1 million (Katz and Hays 2004; Jayawant and Balkrishnan 2005).

The largest single group of OxyContin prescribers became family physicians, who accounted for 21% of all OxyContin prescriptions in 2000 (Tough 2001). It was this rapidly expanded access to the drug, and the fact that many prescribers lacked the training and skill to responsibly prescribe the drug, that was fundamentally linked to the spread of OxyContin abuse (Tough 2001).

The Marketing of OxyContin

The introduction of OxyContin coincided with a fundamental rethinking of how pain should be treated and managed in the field of medicine. For years, terminally ill patients suffered needlessly because doctors resisted prescribing frequent, potent doses of opioids out of the fear that the patients might become addicted. But with new studies showing that pain was a seriously undertreated condition, OxyContin provided a breakthrough opportunity for Purdue Pharma. Until then, the company's bestselling drug was the long-acting oral morphine formulation MS-Contin, which had limited appeal in part because it contained morphine and the stigma that came with it. OxyContin had broader appeal because the active ingredient, oxycodone, did not carry the degree of social stigma of morphine. "If Grandma is placed on morphine, it's like, 'Oh, my God,'" stated Dr. Howard A. Heit, a pain specialist in Fairfax, Virginia, and a Purdue consultant, in an interview with the *New York Times* in 2001, "but if Grandma comes home placed on OxyContin—that was O.K." (Meier and Peterson 2001).

Although oxycodone had been used as a pain medicine for decades, OxyContin differed in two critical ways from the oxycodone formulations that came before it: the drug utilized a time-release formula, and it was provided in much larger doses. The FDA approved OxyContin to treat moderate to severe pain lasting more than a few days. For Robert E. Mitchell, OxyContin proved nothing short of a wonder drug. A victim of Guillain-Barré syndrome, a rare neurological disorder that can cause paralysis, Mitchell said his pain had become so severe he could not walk. But with OxyContin, he could wear shoes and was able to learn to walk again. "To me, it's like a miracle," he said (Meier and Peterson 2001).

Physician-targeted Strategies

Seeing enormous potential in the drug, Purdue conducted an ambitious and aggressive campaign to market and promote OxyContin. To implement its OxyContin campaign, Purdue significantly increased its sales force to market and promote OxyContin to physicians and other health care practitioners. In 1996, Purdue began promoting OxyContin with a sales force of approximately 300 representatives in its Prescription Sales Division. Through a 1996 co-promotion agreement, Abbott Laboratories provided at least another 300 representatives, doubling the sales force devoted to OxyContin. By 2000, Purdue had more than doubled its own internal sales force to 671 thereby significantly increasing the number of physicians to whom it promoted OxyContin. Each Purdue sales representative had a specific sales territory and was responsible for developing a contact list of about 105 to 140 physicians who were already prescribing opioids or who were candidates for prescribing opioids. In 1996, the 300-plus Purdue sales representatives had a total physician call list of approximately 33,400 to 44,500. By 2000, the nearly 700 representatives had a call list of approximately 70,500 to 94,000 physicians. Purdue stated it offered a "better-than-industry-average" salary and sales bonuses to attract top sales representatives and provide incentives to boost sales (USGAO 2003).

In addition to expanding its sales force, Purdue used multiple approaches to market and promote OxyContin. These approaches included expanding its physician speaker bureau and conducting speaker training conferences, sponsoring pain-related educational programs, issuing OxyContin starter coupons for patients' initial prescriptions, sponsoring pain-related websites, advertising OxyContin in medical journals, and distributing OxyContin marketing items to health care professionals (USGAO 2003).

When OxyContin was first marketed, there were no industry or federal guidelines regarding the promotion of prescription drugs. In July 2002, the Pharmaceutical Research and Manufacturers of America (PhRMA) issued voluntary guidelines on how drug companies should market and promote their drugs to health care professionals (PhRMA 2002). In April 2003, the U.S. Department of Health and Human Service's Office of Inspector General issued voluntary guidelines on how drug companies should market and promote their products to federal health care programs. Neither set of guidelines differentiates between the marketing and promotion of controlled versus non-controlled substances (USGAO 2003).

During the first five years of OxyContin's availability, Purdue brought in between 2,000 to 3,000 doctors for three-day retreats in California, Arizona, and Florida. Purdue paid the transportation and hotel costs of doctors to attend weekend meetings to discuss pain management. Doctors were then recruited and paid fees to speak to other doctors at some of the 7,000 "pain management" seminars that Purdue sponsored around the country. Those meetings stressed the importance of aggressively treating pain with potent, long-acting painkillers like OxyContin. Purdue also contributed to foundations supporting research on pain, to pharmacy schools, and to Internet sites aimed at educating consumers. A reporter from the *New York Times* interviewed Dr. Susan Bertrand, who treats chronic pain in Princeton, West Virginia, and became a Purdue speaker. She explained that for her, the research presented to her at a seminar showing the under-treatment of pain was "almost a religious experience" that made her realize how poorly she and other physicians had been trained to deal with the problem. To help rectify this, she states that she gave about a dozen paid lectures sponsored by Purdue. The company also helped her start the Appalachian Pain Foundation, an educational group on pain management (Meier and Peterson 2001).

Although Purdue's marketing campaign quickly began to pay big dividends, some doctors and pharmacists said they became disturbed by the company's sales tactics. "All companies market," Dr. Diane Meier, a pain specialist at the Mount Sinai School of Medicine in New York, told the *New York Times.* "But these people were in your face all the time." Others criticized the way Purdue recruited doctors. "Essentially, they bought the doctors' prescriptions," said Steve Schondelmeyer, a professor of pharmaceutical economics at the University of Minnesota. "It says to consumers that every time you paid for this drug, you sent your doctor to a nice meeting somewhere" (Meier and Peterson 2001).

From the outset of the OxyContin marketing campaign, Purdue promoted the drug to physicians for noncancer pain conditions that stemmed from arthritis, injuries, and chronic diseases, in addition to cancer pain. Purdue directed its sales representatives to focus on the physicians in their sales territories who were high opioid prescribers. This group included cancer and pain specialists, primary care physicians, and physicians who were high prescribers of Purdue's older product, MS-Contin. One of Purdue's goals was to identify primary care physicians who would expand the company's OxyContin prescribing base. Sales representatives were also directed to call on oncology nurses, consultant pharmacists, hospices, hospitals, and nursing homes (USGAO 2003).

From OxyContin's launch until July 2001, Purdue used two key promotional messages for primary care physicians and other high prescribers of opioids. The first was that physicians should prescribe OxyContin for their pain patients both as the drug "to start with and to stay with." The second message contrasted the dosing of other opioid pain relievers with OxyContin dosing as "the hard way versus the easy way" to dose because OxyContin's twice-a-day dosing was more convenient for patients. Purdue's sales representatives promoted OxyContin to physicians as an initial opioid treatment for moderate to severe pain lasting more than a few days, to be prescribed instead of other single-entity opioid analgesics or short-acting combination opioid pain relievers. By 2003, primary care physicians had grown to constitute nearly half of all OxyContin prescribers, based on data from IMS Health (USGAO 2003).

From 1996, when OxyContin was introduced to the market, to July 2002, Purdue had funded more than 20,000 pain-related educational programs through direct sponsorship or financial grants. These grants included support for programs to provide physicians with opportunities to earn required continuing medical education credits, such as grand round presentations at hospitals and medical education seminars at state and local medical conferences (USGAO 2003).

Consumer-targeted Strategies

To reach consumers, Purdue financed an Internet site where OxyContin was promoted, and also contributed to professional advocacy groups. In addition to its corporate website, which provided product information, Purdue established the Partners Against Pain website in 1997 to provide consumers with information about pain management and pain treatment options. According to the FDA, the website also contained information about OxyContin. Separate sections provided information for patients and caregivers, medical professionals, and institutions. This website included a "Find a Doctor" feature to help consumers find physicians who treat pain in their area (USGAO 2003).

Purdue also funded websites such as FamilyPractice.com that offered physicians free continuing medical educational programs on pain management, and contributed to the funding of website development and support for health care groups such as the American Chronic Pain Association and the American Academy of Pain Medicine. In addition, Purdue was one of twenty-eight corporate donors listed on the website of the American Pain Society, the mission of which was to improve pain-related education, treatment, and professional practice. Purdue also sponsored painfullyobvious.com, which it described as a youth-focused "message campaign designed to provide information and stimulate open discussion on the dangers of prescription drug abuse" (USGAO 2003).

In 1999, Purdue provided its sales representatives with 14,000 copies of a promotional video to distribute to physicians. The video, titled *From One Pain Patient to Another: Advice from Patients Who Have Found Relief,* was designed to encourage patients to report their pain and to alleviate concerns about taking opioids. Purdue stated that the video was for use "in physician waiting rooms, as a 'check out' item for an office's patient education library, or as an educational tool for office or hospital staff to utilize with patients and their families" (USGAO 2003).

Additionally, Purdue used a patient starter coupon program for OxyContin to provide patients with a free limited-time prescription. Unlike patient assistance programs, which provide free prescriptions to patients in financial need, a coupon program is intended to enable all patients to try a new drug through a one-time free prescription (USGAO 2003).

The OxyContin marketing message caught on with many doctors who had little experience in prescribing powerful opioids or in treating chronic pain. One result of this was that drug abusers often succeeded in their efforts to feign a pain condition or manipulate the doctor into prescribing OxyContin (Meier and Peterson 2001). Another possible factor contributing to the abuse and diversion of OxyContin was the FDA's original decision to label the drug as having less abuse potential than other oxycodone products because of its controlled-release formulation. FDA officials stated that when OxyContin was approved, the agency believed the controlled-release formulation would result in less abuse potential because, when taken properly, the drug would be absorbed slowly, without providing the rapid, intense drug effect sought by abusers. Additionally, the safety warning on the OxyContin label may also have contributed to the abuse and diversion of the drug by inadvertently giving abusers information on how the drug could be misused. The label warned that the tablets should not be broken, chewed, or crushed because such action could result in the rapid release and absorption of a potentially toxic dose of oxycodone. The FDA places similar safety warnings on other drugs to ensure that they are used properly. Neither FDA officials nor other experts they consulted with anticipated that crushing the controlled-release tablet and injecting or snorting the drug would become widespread and lead to a high level of abuse (USGAO 2003). But perhaps the biggest contributor to the epidemic of abuse and diversion that would soon follow the introduction and meteoric rise in sales of

OxyContin was that word began to spread of just how easy it was to bypass the time-release matrix of the formulation by simply crushing the pill with a spoon, a lighter, even a thumbnail, and that the resulting powder, when snorted or mixed with water and injected, produced a very potent high (Tough 2001).

Table 8.2 summarizes the increase in painkiller market share for moderate to severe pain of OxyContin from 1996 to 2000.

The Unfolding of an Epidemic

The illegal use of OxyContin mushroomed even though, as a DEA schedule II controlled substance, no drug in the United States was more tightly regulated (Meier and Peterson 2001).

Table 8.2

Changing U.S. Market Share of Prescription Opioids
for Moderate to Severe Pain, 1996–2000

1996 Market Share		2000 Market Share	
Fentanyl transdermal	33%	OxyContin	53%
Morphine SR	27%	Fentanyl transdermal	23%
Oxycodone	22%	Oxycodone	10%
OxyContin	10%	Morphine SR	9%
Morphine	9%	Morphine	4%
Hydromorphono	3%	Hydromorphone	1%

(Davis et al. 2003)   SR = sustained release

Abuse of prescription opioids is not new. However, two primary factors set OxyContin abuse apart from other prescription drug abuse. First, OxyContin is a powerful drug that contains a much larger amount of the active ingredient, oxycodone, than other prescription pain relievers. By crushing the tablet and ingesting, snorting, or injecting it, people who abuse the opioid experience its powerful effects rapidly instead of gradually over a twelve-hour period. Second, huge profits could be made in the illegal sale of OxyContin. A 40 mg pill cost approximately $4 by prescription but could be sold for as much as $40 on the street, depending on the area of the country (CSAT 2008).

Reports of OxyContin abuse first surfaced in the rural areas of Maine during the late 1990s and then spread down the East Coast to encompass West Virginia, Kentucky, and southern Ohio. The *Bangor Daily News* was among the very first media sources to report on the drug and its rampant abuse, and included the properties of the drug, methods to bypass the time-release of the drug, tactics used for diversion, and concerns of the medical profession about the potential for abuse (Inciardi and Goode 2003). The areas hardest hit by OxyContin abuse included rural Appalachia and the Ohio valley; Kentucky was one of the leading states for OxyContin-related crime (Inciardi and Goode 2003). Media coverage gained more thrust after Kentucky's "Operation OxyFest 2001." Newspaper headlines heralded stories about the miracle drug OxyContin and how it was abused, and media coverage included stories about robberies, theft, fraud, pharmacy break-ins, and features of several pill mill doctors who supported the addiction of their patients by frequently prescribing the drug. The extensive media coverage and hype seemed to make a "villain" out of OxyContin, and there was a concern that the exhaustive media focus enhanced the popularity of the drug and contributed to its abuse (Jayawant and Balkrishnan 2005). Soon, there was also a corresponding surge in the number of patients presenting to hospitals and substance abuse treatment programs for opioid addiction, the majority of whom were using OxyContin (Jayawant and Balkrishnan 2005).

Susan's Story

Susan came to my office with her mother. She was an 18-year-old high school senior from a small town. She no longer spent time with her family and had stopped most of her extracurricular activities at school. Her boyfriend was in treatment for OxyContin addiction and her mother was concerned because Susan seemed to have a problem as well. She described use of alcohol and marijuana since age fourteen, but it had never been regular, primarily on weekends. She had no problems with school or her family until the past six months. She tried Vicodin about a year ago and liked the effect; it calmed her and gave her more energy. Her boyfriend used more often and supported her experimentation with new opioids. They began to spend more time with a group their age that did opioids regularly. She tried OxyContin by snorting and found it to be the best thing she had ever experienced, until she smoked it. The group she hung out with had started to smoke OxyContin, which resulted in an extremely rapid, powerful high. She got hooked almost immediately and started to use daily. She could not imagine life without it. She spent all of her money on OxyContin and was stealing from her family. She smoked it multiple times a day, at great expense. She said it made her feel fantastic, better than real life, as if she was loved by everyone.

Bill's Story

Bill was 26 when he came to see me. He had been using heroin for the past three months. As a senior in high school, he had experienced a minor injury that had resulted in a prescription of Vicodin for pain. Bill had just begun experimenting with alcohol and marijuana, so he shared the pills with his four best friends. They all liked them and began to seek out doctors willing to prescribe opioids to them. They were able to easily obtain Vicodin, and occasionally OxyContin. They all found OxyContin to be much more desirable, especially when crushed and snorted. He said he "loved it and could not live without it." The five of them continued to party together and use individually. Bill began to buy OxyContin regularly and use it by smoking. He said the high was instantaneous and dramatic. He made a great deal of money working on Alaskan fishing boats all summer. He was unable to obtain or use OxyContin while at sea, but as soon as he returned home he would go right back to it. He smoked OxyContin multiple times a day and had run out of money long before he was to return to Alaska. He was using between 300 mg and 400 mg of OxyContin a day. He collected unemployment, which was not enough to provide for regular OxyContin, but he couldn't stop. To save money he had started to use heroin instead.

Geographic and Economic Factors

Why OxyContin abuse became so rampant across stretches of Appalachia and other rural areas remained an open question. But authorities noted that the prevalence of retirees and mine workers with health care plans and prescription cards invited the exploitation of the elderly and others by illicit brokers involved in the diversion and sale of the drug (Clines and Meier 2001). Many of these same rural areas had economies reliant on labor-intensive industries such as logging or coal mining. These areas had been economically depressed for quite some time, making it tempting for people with legitimate prescriptions to sell them for a profit (CSAT 2008). And according to the DEA, the abuse and diversion of OxyContin in some states may have been a reflection of the geographic area's history of prescription drug abuse. According to a 2001 report by the High Intensity Drug Trafficking Area (HIDTA) program, the Appalachian region, which encompasses parts of Kentucky, Tennessee, Virginia, and West Virginia, had been severely affected by prescription drug abuse, including oxycodone, for many years. Three of the four states—Kentucky, Virginia, and West Virginia—were among the initial states to report OxyContin abuse and diversion. Historically, oxycodone, manufactured under brand names such as Percocet, Percodan, and Tylox, was among the most diverted prescription drugs in Appalachia, and according to the report, OxyContin became the drug of choice in several areas within the region (USGAO 2003).

Hazard, Kentucky, has a long tradition of self-medication. Moonshine and marijuana, grown in its fertile soil, have long helped to blot out depression, boredom, even physical pain. Eastern Kentucky has one of the nation's highest cancer rates, and many residents suffer from chronic mining and timber injuries. OxyContin seemed like the most potent antidote yet to the local despair. "If there's ever been a drug made that will knock depression out for the short term, it's OxyContin," says therapist Mike Spare. "The euphoria sucks you in" (Rosenberg 2001).

Increases in OxyContin-related crime rates were attributed to the increasing number of abusers and the expense of illicit OxyContin. With a street price of roughly $1 per milligram ($80 per pill), drug price became a risk factor for crime related to obtaining the drug (Jayawant and Balkrishnan 2005). Indeed, the high street value of OxyContin fueled the burglary and robbery of pharmacies, and also made OxyContin a very expensive drug habit for those who became addicted to it (Jayawant and Balkrishnan 2005).

Medicaid fraud provided an inexpensive way of obtaining OxyContin to abuse or sell. A Medicaid patient would pay $3 for a bottle of one hundred 80 mg OxyContin tablets (Inciardi and Goode 2003), and in the areas of the country where jobs and money were scarce, OxyContin's high street price was difficult to resist.

Attempts to Control the Epidemic of OxyContin Abuse

Unlike illegal drugs of abuse such as cocaine or heroin, the production, marketing, and distribution of OxyContin are monitored by state and federal health officials. Many of these regulators began trying to figure out how the outbreak occurred and what they might have done to prevent it (Meier and Peterson 2001).

By 2000, the reports of illegal use, misuse, abuse, and diversion of OxyContin prompted federal and state agencies and Purdue to begin taking actions to address the problem. In July 2001, the FDA approved a revised OxyContin label, adding the highest level of safety warning that the FDA can place on an approved drug product. The agency also collaborated with Purdue to develop and implement a risk management plan to help detect and prevent abuse and diversion of OxyContin. Risk management plans were not used at the time OxyContin was approved (USGAO 2003). The FDA cited Purdue Pharma twice for using potentially false or misleading medical journal advertisements for OxyContin in violation of the Food, Drug, and Cosmetic Act of 1938, including one ad that did not include warnings of the potentially fatal risks associated with its use (USGAO 2003; Jayawant and Balkrishnan 2005).

In Virginia, disgruntled OxyContin users and their relatives filed a $5.2 billion class-action lawsuit against Purdue, charging that the company failed to adequately warn consumers of the "uniquely" addictive potential of OxyContin and that it marketed the drug irresponsibly. The lawsuit was intended to include virtually everyone whose life had been adversely affected by the drug. Many of the plaintiffs claimed they became hooked taking OxyContin exactly as their doctors prescribed it. Others were pre-scribed OxyContin when a milder drug would have been sufficient. Even patients and the relatives of users who suffered no ill effects from the drug were encouraged to sign on, claiming a "risk of addiction" (Rosenberg 2001).

West Virginia Attorney General Darrell V. McGraw Jr. filed a similar lawsuit in 2000, charging that Purdue marketed the drug deceptively to treat even minor pain. The state wanted Purdue to fund drug addiction treatment programs and to reimburse insurers for unnecessary prescrip-tions. To bolster his case, McGraw collected anecdotes from doctors who stated that Purdue drug reps tried to strong-arm them by telling them that elderly patients would sue if they refused to prescribe OxyContin to treat common ailments like arthritis. McGraw said that leverage for the threat came from a California jury that had recently ordered a physician to pay $1.5 million for failing to prescribe adequate painkillers, including OxyContin, to a terminally ill cancer patient (Rosenberg 2001).

Purdue Pharma Responds

A spokesman for Purdue Pharma stated that the company was not aware of significant problems with OxyContin abuse until April 2000, when a front-page article in the *Bangor Daily News* claiming that OxyContin "is quickly becoming the recreational drug of choice in Maine" landed on the desk of Purdue's senior medical director, Dr. J. David Haddox. Later that summer, Purdue formed a response team consisting of medical personnel, public relations specialists, and two of the company's top executives, which guided the company's OxyContin campaign from that time forward (Tough 2001).

Purdue officials expressed surprise that OxyContin could be abused. Haddox stated he thought the time-release formula would make the pill "less desirable to addicts." Later in 2000, Purdue formed a focus group of twenty consultants to explore methods for doctors to better identify potential drug abusers. Purdue also began having its sales force remind doctors that drugs like OxyContin "are common targets for both drug abusers and drug addicts." Purdue began planning to reformulate OxyContin to make it less appealing to abusers. The company also began to educate students on the dangers of prescription drugs (Meier and Peterson 2001).

Purdue Pharma, acutely aware of the negative publicity surrounding OxyContin, began working furiously to protect its $1.5 billion brand with additional actions and initiatives (Adler 2003). Steps were taken to reduce the potential for abuse of OxyContin and other pain medications. Its website lists the following initiatives:

- funding educational programs to teach health care professionals how to assess and treat patients suffering from pain
- providing prescribers with tamper-proof prescription pads
- developing and distributing more than one million brochures to pharmacists and health care professionals to help educate them about medication diversion
- working with health care and law enforcement officials to address prescription drug abuse
- endorsing the development of state and national prescription drug monitoring programs to detect diversion

In addition, the company was attempting to research and develop other pain management products that would be more resistant to abuse and diversion. The company estimated that it would take significant time for such products to be brought to market (CSAT 2008).

Purdue's executives saw the company as an unwitting victim of criminal activity, which they compared to the story of Johnson & Johnson in 1982 when seven people were killed by Extra-Strength Tylenol tablets that had been laced with cyanide. The critics of Purdue preferred to compare its practices with those of the tobacco companies, who were increasingly likely to be found liable for deaths caused by their products (Tough 2001).

Eventually, Purdue agreed to pay $19.5 million to twenty-six states and the District of Columbia to settle complaints that it encouraged physicians to overprescribe OxyContin. One of the sticking points in the complaints made by state attorneys general was that the company urged doctors to prescribe OxyContin every eight hours instead of the twelve-hour dose approved by the FDA. The company also agreed to stop basing bonuses for its sales staff solely on the volume of OxyContin prescribed (Associated Press 2007).

The lack of coordination between Purdue and the government agencies that regulate it had serious fallout for the afflicted communities, as local police, small-town mayors, and individual doctors and pharmacies were forced to create their own policies to contain the epidemic. Six states— Florida, Maine, Vermont, West Virginia, Ohio, and South Carolina— introduced regulations to make it more difficult for Medicaid recipients to receive OxyContin. Following a rash of pharmacy robberies in the Boston area, dozens of drugstores in Massachusetts pulled OxyContin from their shelves, only to be ordered by the state pharmacy board to resume carrying the drug. In Pulaski, Virginia, police began a program requiring patients picking up OxyContin prescriptions from local pharmacies to be fingerprinted, a development that alarmed civil liberties organizations. Doctors in many states, sometimes fearing reprisals from the DEA, refused to prescribe OxyContin even to patients clearly in need (Tough 2001).

Hospitals also began taking new approaches to address the problem of prescription opiate abuse. Mercy Hospital in Portland, Maine, gave OxyContin patients urine screens to verify that they were not taking too much, or that they were taking the drug when prescribed and not selling it on the street. A Cincinnati-based hospital chain, the Health Alliance, decided to limit OxyContin to just a few types of patients, such as those with cancer, after determining that another painkiller would be just as effective, cheaper, and less prone to abuse (Meier and Peterson 2001).

Around the time of media reports of widespread OxyContin abuse, Purdue began a national campaign to inform the public that it was doing everything possible to combat the problem and to make sure that only patients with legitimate needs received the drug. However, there were reports in the media of inconsistent effort on the part of Purdue to curtail the widespread abuse of its product (Meier 2001).

As reported in the *New York Times* in December 10, 2001, Myrtle Beach, South Carolina, was a major hot spot of OxyContin abuse, with one clinic being especially problematic. Some pharmacists and a law enforcement official warned Purdue of the activity at the clinic but apparently the company did little, if anything, about it. The drug of choice at the clinic was OxyContin. Purdue Pharma's own records stated that the year's first-quarter sales of OxyContin in a sales territory that included Myrtle Beach grew by more than $1 million. During the same period, sales in the territory with the next-biggest growth in the country grew by $700,000. Federal officials said the drug maker should have investigated whether the surge in the Myrtle Beach territory was caused by physicians overprescribing the drug or by people misusing it. "There was total disregard for what was going on over there," said Cheri Crowley, the federal Drug Enforcement Administration agent in charge of the agency's investigation into the clinic (Meier 2001).

Purdue Pharma, as well as some doctors, began to worry that the extensive media coverage of OxyContin abuse was scaring away patients who needed the drug. "The publicity, of which you are a part, is causing patients to call us in tears because their physicians are taking them off therapy," said Robin Hogen, a company spokesman. "This is becoming a sad case of patients being abused by drug abusers" (Meier and Peterson 2001).

The Aftermath

Analysis of the extensive media coverage of OxyContin abuse and diversion later revealed that some of the reports were exaggerated or unfounded (Libby 2005). The DEA launched an aggressive campaign against OxyContin in February 2001 in response to sharp criticism the agency received from the General Accounting Office over its failure to decrease the illegal drug supply in the United States despite a thirty-year effort and billions of dollars, and over the alleged pervasiveness of OxyContin abuse (Libby 2008; Libby 2005).

Physician practice has been altered by the threat of investigation and prosecution. Ziegler and Lovrich (2003) conducted a study investigating whether the fear of prosecution among physicians prescribing opioids was warranted, and if so, what factors contributed to its likelihood. As part of their research, the authors interviewed chief prosecutors in four states regarding their knowledge and attitudes on the legitimate prescribing of opioid painkillers. The study, published in 2003, found that almost 75% of the prosecutors surveyed believed that simply taking prescription opioids posed a moderate or high risk of addiction. A little less than half of prosecutors surveyed said they would recommend that the police begin an investigation merely on the basis of evidence that a physician was prescribing high doses of opioids to some patients for more than a month (Ziegler and Lovrich 2003; Szalavitz 2004).

CHAPTER 9

Twelve Step Programs for Opioid Abuse

Twelve Step programs specific to opioid abuse and dependence include Narcotics Anonymous (NA) and Methadone Anonymous (MA) and are modeled after Alcoholics Anonymous (AA). AA is widely considered the most successful treatment for alcoholism and has helped millions of alcoholics achieve sobriety. The Twelve Step model emphasizes acceptance of addiction as a chronic, progressive disease that can be arrested through abstinence but not cured (NA 2010). Elements of the Twelve Step model include spiritual growth, personal responsibility, and helping other addicts. By inducing a shift in the consciousness of the addict, Twelve Step programs offer a holistic solution and are also a resource for emotional support (Humphreys et al. 2004).

Twelve Step groups for drug abusers share the following characteristics (Hawkins 1980):

1. Participation in the group is voluntary.

2. Members share a common drug use problem.

3. The primary purpose of meeting together is for members to deal with their shared problem.

4. Members provide help and support to each other.

5. The help and support process involves face-to-face interaction.

6. Members are responsible for and have control of the group.

7. Open sharing of information occurs in the group (that is, there is no censorship of discussion).

8. The group performs an advocacy function.

9. The group provides a formal explanation or ideology concerning the members' shared problem.

10. The group is not professionally supported.

Accepting drug addiction as a chronic and relapsing disorder has helped professionals better understand the vital role played by Twelve Step programs. Twelve Step programs are not considered treatment, nor are they intended as substitutes for treatment. Rather, they are mutual help organizations that provide ongoing and indefinite support as members work toward achieving and then maintaining abstinence, as well as general personal growth and character development (Chappel and DuPont 1999).

NA and MA are effective in part because they provide competition and an alternative to drug use. Involvement in Twelve Step programs can improve a member's social support and social network, a potentially highly reinforcing aspect the person stands to lose if he or she resumes using drugs. Other reinforcing elements of Twelve Step involvement include recognition for increasingly longer periods of abstinence and frequent awareness of the consequences of drug and alcohol use through attendance of meetings (Higgins 1997). Research shows that when people develop a pattern of Twelve Step program attendance early in treatment, they tend to stay involved as they gain time in recovery; thus, the therapist should emphasize and facilitate early Twelve Step program involvement (Weiss et al. 2000).

Narcotics Anonymous

Narcotics Anonymous (NA) is the oldest, largest, and best known of the Twelve Step fellowships addressing recovery from opioid and other drug addiction.

The idea for creating a Twelve Step program specifically to help drug addicts had emerged several times before the official founding of NA in 1953. In early 1947, a group of drug addicts began to meet as part of a treatment center in Lexington Federal Prison in Lexington, Kentucky. This group was based on the Twelve Steps of AA and called itself NARCO or Addicts Anonymous. The group continued to meet weekly for more than twenty years. In 1948, one of the graduates from the NARCO program moved to New York City and started a similar group in the New York Prison System. This was the first group to use the name Narcotics Anonymous. The group dissolved soon after it was founded but similar, independent groups simultaneously appeared in other parts of the United States, suggesting a strong unmet need for such an organized program (Laudet 2008; Zafiridis 2001).

Narcotics Anonymous was founded as AANA in Los Angeles in 1953, with most of the founding members having achieved their clean time from opioids through AA. This group differed from its predecessors in that it specifically attempted to form a mutual help group. The first documented meeting of AANA occurred August 17, 1953. In September of that year, AA granted the group permission to use the AA Steps and Traditions but not the AA name. At this point the organization officially changed its name to Narcotics Anonymous, or NA. The first NA publication was issued in 1954 and was called the *Little Yellow Booklet*. It contained the Twelve Steps and early drafts of several pieces that would be included in subsequent program literature (Laudet 2008).

The initial NA group had trouble finding places that would allow members to meet and often had to meet in people's homes. The state of New York was one of the most difficult places for NA to get off the ground because the Rockefeller drug laws made it a crime for drug addicts to gather together for any reason, effectively making NA illegal. Addicts had to resort to cruising around the vicinity of meeting places and checking for surveillance to make sure the meetings were not being monitored by law enforcement. The meetings became known as "bunny meetings" as members "hopped" from place to place to avoid being detected by the police (Laudet 2008).

Following a period of instability that included several months in 1959 when no meetings were held, the founding members dedicated themselves to restarting NA. In the early 1960s, meetings began to form again and grow. The basic text of NA, called the *White Booklet,* was written in 1962 and became the backbone of NA meetings and the NA program. NA was dubbed by some a "hip pocket program" because the entire literature could be carried in a member's hip pocket. The *White Booklet* was expanded and republished in 1966 as the *NA White Book,* and the first NA phone line was established and opened in 1960.

Another important milestone in NA's development was the forming of the first "H&I" (hospitals and institutions) subcommittee in 1963. The H&I carries the NA recovery message into institutions, such as hospitals and prisons, to serve people who cannot attend Twelve Step meetings on the outside. Also that year a Parent Service Board (later renamed the World Service Board) was formed to monitor and preserve organization integrity. NA grew slowly during the 1960s as it learned what was and was not effective and helpful, as relapse rates and friction between NA groups began to decrease. During the 1970s, NA began a period of dramatic growth, in part coinciding with a social context in the United States in which drug use had become more accepted and less stigmatized. In 1970, there were only twenty regular, weekly meetings throughout the United States. Within two years, the movement spread to Europe and Australia, and has continued to grow into a worldwide organization.

The first edition of the *NA Basic Text* was published in 1983, which contributed to NA's tremendous growth; the sixth edition was published in 2008 (Laudet 2008; NA 2010). Currently, NA is well established throughout much of the Americas, western Europe, Australia, the Middle East, New Zealand, and Eastern Europe. Newly formed groups and NA communities can be found scattered throughout the Indian subcontinent, Africa, and East Asia. The organization is a worldwide multilingual, multicultural fellowship with more than 50,000 weekly meetings in 130 countries. NA books and literature are currently available in thirty-six languages, with translations in process for sixteen additional languages (NA 2010).

The Program of NA

One of the biggest factors driving the founding of NA, as well as other later specialized Twelve Step organizations, was that AA discouraged its drug-addicted members from speaking of their drug addiction. This attitude of some AA meetings is reflected in the AA principle of "singleness of purpose" and is expressed in a statement read at the introduction of some AA meetings that states "in keeping with AA's singleness of purpose, please limit your sharing to alcohol." Thus, people attending AA who do not identify alcohol as their primary problem may not be able to maximally benefit from Twelve Step groups where alcohol and alcoholism is the primary topic of conversation. Another vitally important aspect of successful involvement and participation in a Twelve Step program is *identification with peers* who seek a solution to a shared problem. The experiences of individuals dependent on drugs are likely to differ significantly from those of alcoholics (Laudet 2008). However, these limitations to the AA program have dramatically diminished, as people with multiple addictions are now the norm in AA and such conversations are commonplace in most major metropolitan area AA meetings.

The approach of NA and other Twelve Step groups is non-professional and is based on mutual help. The primary therapeutic value stems from addicts helping other addicts, and the power of the process that occurs in these groups in helping the addict achieve recovery has been repeatedly documented in the published research (Kooyman 1993; Yablonsky 1994; Yablonsky 1969; Zafiridis 2001). During an NA meeting, each member shares his or her personal experiences and seeks help from people who have lived through similar situations and found a way out. Attendance at NA groups is open to anyone regardless of religion or lack thereof, socioeconomic status, gender, or nationality, and the only prerequisite is a desire to stop using drugs. NA involvement is also open to people who suffer from psychiatric illness in addition to drug abuse (Laudet 2008). An important statement regarding membership is provided on the NA website: "NA as a whole has no opinion on outside issues, including prescribed medications. Use of psychiatric medication and other medically indicated drugs prescribed by a physician and taken under medical supervision is not seen as compromising a person's recovery in NA."

NA applies the disease model to drug abuse and addiction, which involves the recognition that addiction is a relapsing illness requiring total abstinence (Luty 2003). Central to the NA program is the concept of a *spiritual awakening,* emphasizing its practical value not its philosophical or metaphysical import (NA 1992).

Another key component of NA is the sponsorship relationship. A sponsor is an older member of an NA group who helps a new member work through the Twelve Steps and otherwise provides support; sponsors play a key role in helping many NA members achieve sobriety (NA 1992). Research has demonstrated that working with a sponsor significantly decreases the risk of relapse (Sheeren 1988; Isenhart 1997). The activities carried out by the sponsor are beneficial not only to the newer member but also to the sponsors themselves; Cross and colleagues (1990) found that in a ten-year follow-up, 91% of NA members who became sponsors had maintained their sobriety. Another possible explanation of why NA and other Twelve Step programs are effective comes from the therapeutic value of solidarity, commitment, and caring for others identified by humanistic and existential psychologists such as Viktor Frankl (Laudet 2008).

Research on NA

Although research on effectiveness and patient outcome in NA and MA is limited, AA research has revealed success in maintaining abstinence. Some studies examining participants in AA and NA found that meeting attendance was linked with abstinence, freedom from substance use problems, freedom from significant distress and psychiatric problems, and increased employment (Ouimette, Moos, and Finney 1998). Many prominent addiction researchers emphasize the important role that ongoing involvement in Twelve Step programs plays in recovery (Chappel and DuPont 1999).

The anonymity of NA (as with AA), as well as other factors, has precluded randomized controlled trials comparing the effectiveness of NA either to other types of therapy or recovery programs, or to no therapy or recovery program at all. Despite this limitation in the scientific investigation of NA's effectiveness, several studies reveal important information about how NA helps members abstain from opiates and other drugs.

The first longitudinal follow-up study investigating the impact of NA involvement on new members was published in 2003 by Toumbourou and Hamilton. The researchers interviewed and followed ninety-one new NA members. The strongest factor in predicting continued abstinence from substance use was higher levels of service work in NA. Service work in this study included chairing a meeting, helping in-service positions, being sponsored, and sponsoring others. The study also found that regular and stable NA group attendance was associated with Step work (completing Steps Three to Ten), improvements in social support (perceived friendship benefits, less social isolation, finding a spouse or partner), and an approximate fourfold reduction in drug use. The authors also found NA to be underutilized and suggested that future research focus on identifying barriers to NA participation.

Improvement in psychological functioning as a result of NA involvement has been observed by Christo and Sutton (1994). Among the two hundred NA members in their study, those who had been off drugs and involved with NA for longer periods tended to have lower anxiety and higher self-esteem, with those abstinent over three years exhibiting levels of anxiety and self-esteem similar to those of a comparison group (Christo and Sutton 1994).

Serving as an NA sponsor over a one-year period was strongly linked with substantial improvements in abstinence, suggesting that the process of providing direction and support to other addicts strengthens one's own recovery (Crape et al. 2002).

Spiritual beliefs and endorsement of the disease concept are not prerequisites for NA membership; neither were spiritual beliefs found to cause previous drug use or possible future relapses (Christo and Franey 1995).

Another study (Vederhus and Kristensen 2006) examining the effectiveness of Twelve Step programs surveyed patients two years after treatment. A total of 114 patients who started attending NA and/or AA after treatment were sent surveys. Of these, 65 patients returned the survey and 10 other patients were interviewed by phone. The authors found that 38% of the respondents participated in Twelve Step programs two years after treatment; among these regular participants, 81% had been abstinent during the previous six months, compared with only 26% of those who had stopped attending Twelve Step meetings. The likelihood of being drug free was 12.6 times higher for those who participated regularly in Twelve Step meetings than for those who did not. Also, people who dropped out of Twelve Step programs had more severe psychiatric conditions than those who continued. It should be noted that involvement in NA was not compared with involvement in AA.

Methadone Anonymous

The catalyst of Methadone Anonymous (MA) occurred in 1991 when a staff member of a methadone maintenance clinic in Baltimore attended an NA meeting and observed a woman receive an "Anniversary Chip" in recognition of clean time from heroin, only to be told to return the chip when she shared that methadone maintenance helped make it possible. This staff person went on to develop a Twelve Step program for methadone maintenance treatment (MMT) patients (MA 2007a).

MA believes "that methadone is a therapeutic tool of recovery that may or may not be discontinued in time, dependent upon the needs of the individual" and that continued abstinence from opioids and other chemicals, including alcohol, is the foremost goal of recovery. Most MA meetings are hosted by MMT clinics, and there are at least six hundred MA chapters worldwide (MA 2007b).

There are very few published studies involving MA. However, one study found that, similar to members of other Twelve Step programs, MA members undergo a spiritually mediated transformation in their recovery process, with members describing methadone as the core of the group experience and an aid to spiritual transformation (Glickman et al. 2006). Length of time in MA has been linked with reductions in the use of alcohol, cocaine, and marijuana. Clients in methadone maintenance programs have rated components of MA to be significantly more helpful to recovery than methadone maintenance treatment program (MMTP) components, suggesting that MA participation has benefits not available in professionally driven MMTPs (Gilman, Galanter, and Dermatis 2001).

Pills Anonymous

Pills Anonymous (PA) is a Twelve Step fellowship for those seeking recovery from addiction to prescription drugs, including prescription opioids.

Membership is open to anyone with a desire to stop using prescription drugs. The fellowship advocates "complete abstinence from prescription drugs, alcohol, all medication taken not as prescribed, as well as all other mind-altering substances" (PA 2010). Very little has been written about PA in the published research.

Twelve Step Programs for Special Populations

Twelve Step recovery programs promote abstinence from all mind-altering substances, and although the World Services of each fellowship do not promote an opinion on the use of prescribed medications, people who need medications to manage psychiatric symptoms or opioid dependence may not feel welcomed at some traditional Twelve Step meetings, because some members misinterpret the use of medications as not being abstinent. The unfortunate result is that individuals in need of support and involvement with Twelve Step groups feel discouraged and unwelcome. In response, new Twelve Step organizations have developed specifically to offer recovery support to people who are dually diagnosed with a substance use disorder and a mental illness, and for individuals receiving methadone maintenance for opiate dependence (Laudet 2008).

Double Trouble in Recovery

Double Trouble in Recovery (DTR) was started in New York in 1989 and has more than two hundred groups meeting in fourteen states, with the largest number in New York and growing memberships in Georgia, Colorado, New Mexico, and New Jersey. New DTR groups begin at the initiative of consumers or professionals who believe that Twelve Step fellowships are a useful addition to formal treatment. DTR developed as a grassroots initiative and functions with minimal involvement from the professional community. Groups meet in psychosocial clubs; supported residences for mental health clients; day-treatment programs for mental health, substance abuse, and dual-diagnosis clients; and hospital inpatient units and community-based organizations. All DTR groups are led by people in recovery (Vogel et al. 1998).

One survey found that DTR members' primary problem substances were cocaine and alcohol, and the most prevalent psychiatric diagnoses were schizophrenia (43%), bipolar disorder (25%), and unipolar depression (26%) (Laudet et al. 2000). The DTR website (www.doubletroubleinrecovery.org) states that 76% of DTR members receive a prescribed regimen of psychiatric medication, which they consider a critical part of the dually diagnosed client's recovery process, as is abstinence from drugs and alcohol. DTR also emphasizes the importance of sponsorship.

Dual Recovery Anonymous

Dual Recovery Anonymous (DRA) began in Kansas City in 1989. DRA meetings can be found in most U.S. states as well as in Canada, Australia, New Zealand, India, and Iceland (Laudet 2008).

Worldwide Acceptance

The Twelve Step recovery model was developed in the United States and has become widespread in American culture and the health care delivery system. Unlike other countries such as Australia and most of Western Europe, the United States has adopted an abstinence-based response to drug dependence, making Twelve Step recovery an ideal recovery resource and aftercare model. Interestingly, even in countries where a harm-reduction approach is more typical than a total abstinence approach to addiction, such as Australia, the majority of people with a chronic history of polysubstance abuse choose abstinence from all mood-altering substances as their personal recovery goal. They also report Twelve Step participation patterns that do not significantly differ from their counterparts in the United States (Laudet and Storey 2006; Laudet 2008).

CHAPTER 10

Treatment of Prescription Opioid Addiction

Opioid addiction is the oldest drug addiction and has been treated for centuries, usually by discontinuing use of opioids "cold turkey," as the heroin addicts call it when they are withdrawing with goose bumps all over their bodies. Fortunately, we now know that detoxification is only the first step in the treatment of addiction and has little effect on long-term abstinence when it is not followed by actual addiction treatment. The treatment of prescription opioid addiction is based on the treatment of heroin addiction. Perhaps this is as it should be, for we are discussing the same category of drugs—opioids. However, there are differences that need to be accounted for, and at this time no standardized guidelines for the treatment of prescription opioid addiction exist. The primary treatments for prescription opioid addiction are

- maintenance, with methadone or buprenorphine
- receptor blockade, with naltrexone
- abstinence, primarily a Twelve Step approach

There are an estimated 1 million opioid addicts in the United States and approximately 260,000 receive maintenance treatment; it is the largest treatment intervention for this disease (SAMHSA 2007b). Opioid addiction treatment admissions have escalated with the growing use of prescription opioids. In the past decade, according to SAMHSA's Treatment Episode Data Set (TEDS) report, opioid addiction treatment admissions have increased from 16% to 20% of all treatment admissions (SAMHSA 2010).

Prescription opioid addicts are receiving treatments that are available for heroin, not necessarily specifically developed and proven effective for their drug of choice. Although this is not entirely problematic, it does reveal a lack of data specific to this type of addiction. Some data examining specific treatments for this population are available and will be used to describe the recognized treatment models. There are some comparative studies that examine and compare outcomes among the medications, but not among the main treatments offered. Thus, comparisons using diverse studies and reports must suffice until the data are developed. Bias pervades this field, as do individual approaches. Currently the National Institute on Drug Abuse (NIDA) is funding the Prescription Opioid Addiction Treatment Study (POATS), which is proposed to determine if outcomes can be improved by using both individual drug counseling and buprenorphine/naloxone with standard medical management. It will add to the literature, but is limited to comparing those on buprenorphine who receive counseling to those who are on the medication but do not receive counseling. This study will help advance our understanding of the treatment of prescription opioid addiction, but does not examine the spectrum of treatments available, nor does it compare them all.

The lack of data results in a lack of consensus and thus controversy and differences of opinion. The dramatic increase in use of these substances, with increased death rates and increased treatment utilization, has focused much more attention to the treatment of prescription opioid addiction, and this will drive research, information, and data for use by clinicians. Currently most treatment programs use their basic model, whatever it may be, to address prescription opioids. People with prescription opioid addiction are being treated in methadone maintenance programs, by individual physicians providing buprenorphine or naltrexone, and in abstinence-based residential and outpatient treatment programs. Unfortunately, the prescription opioid addict suffers when research is lacking and the field is not aligned.

Types of Treatment

Methadone Maintenance

Methadone maintenance has been proven to be an effective treatment of heroin addiction, and analyses have suggested removing barriers to access and use (Dole 1972; Rettig and Yarmolinsky 1995; NIH 1997). Long-term treatment of opioid addiction was based on early research revealing long-standing evidence of "altered physiologic function" considered to be protracted abstinence or protracted withdrawal symptoms (Himmelsbach 1942; Martin and Jasinski 1969). These studies supported later decisions to use maintenance medication to limit the physiologic evidence of extended withdrawal and to eliminate craving, thus decreasing the risk of relapse. Dole and Nyswander (1967) suggested altered brain function prior to the discovery of mu-opioid receptors, referring to altered "metabolic" function. The success of methadone maintenance is well documented; it has been shown to block the euphoria associated with heroin and relieve the lengthy abstinence symptoms (Dole 1972; Kosten 1990). Methadone maintenance has also proven to be effective in facilitating psychosocial stabilization, increasing treatment retention, and reducing criminal activity and the risk of infectious disease, especially HIV (Dole 1972; Cooper et al. 1983; Hartel et al. 1989). Despite the evidence of benefits, controversy related to the use of a potentially addictive medication—methadone—to treat opioid addiction remains a subject of discussion among physicians, patients, the general public, and even those working in the addiction field.

Description

Methadone is an opioid agonist and has the potential for addiction, but tolerance develops fairly rapidly and those using a single dose, over time, do not become intoxicated from its use. Methadone is used at methadone maintenance programs that are highly regulated. These programs require daily attendance to obtain medication for months to years. This is a tremendous inconvenience for those on long-term treatment, but it effectively structures the initial involvement and helps to limit diversion of the medication. Dosage is directly related to response and although initial studies tended to use 60 mg, it is more common to use between 100 and

200 mg on a daily basis. The clinics are required to provide psychosocial treatment in addition to the medication, and some are much better at this than others. Methadone programs are often found in inner-city locations, serving an inner-city heroin addict population. Although this is a challenging population to work with, positive outcomes have been achieved with maintenance treatments and little else.

Pros

Methadone is effective in reducing use of heroin. It is also useful in reducing the use of opioids, reducing craving, improving psychosocial stabilization, improving treatment retention, decreasing criminal behavior, and decreasing infectious disease (Dole 1972; Kosten 1990; Cooper et al. 1983; Hartel et al. 1989). Research on methadone treatment of prescription opioid addiction is not as plentiful as that for heroin. There is tremendous overlap, in that most heroin users also use prescribed opioids. Prescription opioid users tend to be Caucasian, are less likely to have a history of intravenous use (although one-third reported injecting), are younger, and are more likely to have pain. Prescription opioid use is highly likely in a methadone maintenance population (Rosenblum et al. 2007). Methadone is effective, inexpensive, and widely used for treatment of heroin addiction and prescription opioid addiction. It is available in most metropolitan areas, but not in all states. It is well tolerated with few side effects. Studies show that there is a high relapse rate in heroin addicts who stop using methadone, up to 80% to 90%, justifying long-term use (McLellan 1983; Ball and Ross 1991; Magura and Rosenblum 2001; Mattick et al. 2003).

Cons

Negative attitudes about methadone, even among physicians and addiction treatment professionals, limit referrals and support stigma about this effective treatment. The clinics are highly regulated—in fact more so than any other aspect of medical care—contributing to stigma and obstacles to ease of use and access by patients. It is very difficult and expensive to go to a clinic daily to pick up medication. The psychosocial therapies are often limited at methadone clinics and, if available, the counseling personnel are often inexperienced or lack adequate training. Diversion of methadone is uncommon, only 4% of street opioids are diverted from methadone clinics (ASAM 2009). The rates of use of other substances while people are on methadone are high, initially 20% to 50% using cocaine and 25% to 40% using alcohol (ASAM 2009). Early treatment termination is a common problem in methadone maintenance programs. Many of these programs are for-profit entities and some provide medication but little else, adding to the stigma associated with methadone maintenance. Those programs serving the underprivileged are losing funding in many states as financial support of social services has been undermined. Reduced funding usually results in loss of the psychosocial treatments. Prescription opioid addicts from higher socioeconomic levels may avoid methadone for a number of reasons, including stigma, exposure to an inner-city population, and exposure to heroin addicts.

Side Effects

The worst possibility, and an increasing problem, is overdose and death, which is the result of respiratory depression. Overdose usually occurs in those naïve to opioids or as the result of inexperienced physicians. This problem is primarily found among prescription opioid users and also among patients receiving methadone for pain, but much less often among patients on methadone maintenance treatment. Relapse to opioid use while on methadone can also result in overdose. Hypogonadism and alteration of normal cardiac function are significant, but rare side effects. Common problems include constipation, sweating, drowsiness, decreased libido, and decreased sexual performance.

Unanswered Questions

Research is needed to answer multiple questions about the use of methadone for prescription opioid addiction:

- Is it effective for prescription opioid addiction? (It is certainly being used for this purpose.)
- Which prescription opioid addicts should be provided methadone maintenance therapy and for how long?
- Is it a good therapy for all opioid addicts, or just for a subgroup?

- Can we identify a genetic variant of the mu-opioid receptor or some other marker to help in this decision making?
- Can people benefit from involvement in both maintenance therapy and Twelve Step programs?

A Reasonable Approach

From a clinical perspective, one is faced with the above questions on a daily basis when dealing with prescription opioid addiction. As a result, some general guidelines, without the benefit of great data, are in order. In general, I would use buprenorphine instead of methadone, but it can be useful and effective in this population. It is reasonable to use methadone for prescription opioid addiction in those who have a long history of addiction, a history of heroin addiction, and especially for those with a history of regular, intravenous use. I also consider it for chronic prescription opioid addiction and for those with multiple relapses. It is inexpensive, so better for those without means or insurance.

Caregivers also have the opportunity to provide leadership in their communities regarding the stigma of maintenance treatments and should always educate and advocate for appropriate treatment with patients, family members, other providers, and the community at large. Opioid addicts who use a maintenance therapy and become actively involved in long-term treatment and Twelve Step programs should be considered for detoxification and abstinence-based treatment.

Buprenorphine Maintenance

Buprenorphine maintenance has been studied extensively for the treatment of heroin dependence and has been shown to be safe and effective for use in office-based settings and to have comparable outcomes to methadone maintenance (Walsh and Preston 1995; Lange 1990; Huestis et al. 1999). Studies examining buprenorphine maintenance for prescription opioid dependence are limited, but enough data are available to reach some general conclusions. It seems that more prescription opioid addicts seek buprenorphine than methadone. A study comparing patients with heroin and prescription opioid dependencies in a primary care office found those using prescription opioids to be younger and have fewer years of opioid use, less treatment history, and less likelihood of hepatitis C history. They were more likely to be white and earn more income. They stayed in treatment longer and had fewer opioid positive urine drug screen tests. The prescription opioid dependent patients had better overall outcomes (Moore et al. 2007). Most prescription opioid users I have treated were very knowledgeable about buprenorphine and the vast majority of those under age 35 years had purchased it on the street for getting by when other opioids were unavailable or to attempt to detoxify themselves.

Description

Buprenorphine is a partial mu agonist, with a slow onset and long duration of action. It is usually provided in a single daily dose, but some people rapidly metabolize it and need at least twice-daily dosing. A partial mu agonist does not completely stimulate the mu-opioid receptors, and as a result buprenorphine is described as having a ceiling effect. Above 32 mg, it does not continue to produce greater opioid effects. Thus, people cannot continue to escalate their dose and become increasingly intoxicated. The ceiling effect is also protective in overdose compared to opioid agonists and seldom results in death by respiratory depression. Respiratory depression and death have been described when buprenorphine has been used in combination with high-dose benzodiazepines or alcohol. It is used to detoxify opioid addicts and for maintenance treatment of opioid addiction. It can be purchased for treatment of pain by injection under the name Buprenex, which is not approved for use in addiction.

Pros

Buprenorphine maintenance has been shown to be as effective as methadone maintenance for the treatment of heroin dependence (Walsh and Preston 1995; Lange 1990; Huestis et al. 1999). However, methadone was shown to be better at retaining heroin addicts in treatment. The preliminary data suggest that buprenorphine maintenance is effective for prescription opioid addiction as well (Moore et al. 2007; Magura et al. 2007). Buprenorphine prescriptions are provided in the privacy of a physician's office for use at home, unlike methadone, which must be taken at the clinic. When patients transition from their opioid of choice to buprenorphine, they usually feel very good and readily begin therapy. Respiratory depression with the risk of fatal overdose is remarkably less likely with buprenorphine than with opioid agonists (Dahan 2006), requiring the addition of other sedatives such as alcohol or benzodiazepines to result in respiratory depression. Buprenorphine is less likely than methadone to alter cardiac function (Wedam et al. 2007) and is less likely to cause the cognitive deficits often seen in early use of methadone (Rapeli et al. 2007). People are much less likely to divert buprenorphine/naloxone (Suboxone) than methadone. Due to the ceiling effect of buprenorphine, it is not very desirable for intoxication, especially among those with significant tolerance to opioids (Walsh and Preston 1995). Overall, opioid addicts using buprenorphine maintenance had less opioid use and decreased craving, much as with methadone (Ling, Rawson, and Compton 1994; Ling et al. 1998; Bickel and Amass 1995).

Cons

If buprenorphine is started too early in opioid withdrawal, it can precipitate sudden, significant opioid withdrawal, called precipitated withdrawal (CSAT 2004a). Buprenorphine has a high affinity for the opioid receptors and effectively kicks off most other opioids, which can result in precipitated opioid withdrawal rather than relief of withdrawal symptoms as intended by using it for detoxification. This occurs when it is administered too early during opioid withdrawal. For those I've detoxified who have used buprenorphine for long periods, at least several months, for maintenance or other reasons, it can be a difficult medication to discontinue, even using a detoxification taper. Withdrawal symptoms can linger for long periods with evidence of minor opioid withdrawal—usually low energy, anxiety, and sleep disturbance. In this way it seems somewhat similar to methadone. It is much more difficult to discontinue than was originally thought. The sublingual absorption has considerable variability among patients, making standardized dosing somewhat difficult (McAleer et al. 2003). Due to the ceiling effect, buprenorphine may not be as effective as methadone for those with very high-dose opioid use. Buprenorphine is available in the privacy of a physician's office, but many physicians provide prescriptions and nothing more—no psychosocial treatment—and do not require it. Buprenorphine is expensive, especially compared to methadone. It is not covered by some insurance plans and many state treatment programs. Buprenorphine is abused, which has been noted wherever it has been provided. It has become a regular drug of abuse in some parts of Europe, but primarily the Subutex formulation. However, most of the misuse noted in one U.S. study was not for intoxication, but for self-treatment of withdrawal (Aitken, Higgs, and Hellard 2008; Hakansson et al. 2007; Cicero, Surratt, and Inciardi 2007). It can be easily obtained from physicians and sold to obtain money for buying other, more desirable opioids.

Side Effects

Buprenorphine itself is unlikely to cause death, but has caused lethal overdose, primarily when injected in combination with high-dose benzodiazepines (Kintz 2001). It can cause respiratory depression when combined with other sedatives, including benzodiazepines and alcohol. Accidental ingestion by children has been reported and is of concern requiring medical consultation, but most often is inconsequential (Hayes, Klein-Schwartz, and Doyon 2008). Many drug interactions occur with buprenorphine due to its metabolism by the cytochrome P450 3A4 enzyme system in the liver (CSAT 2004a). This has to be taken into account when prescribing buprenorphine for people using other medications, especially those used for HIV. The primary side effects of buprenorphine match those of other opioids: nausea, vomiting, constipation, dysphoria, and miosis (pinpoint pupils).

Unanswered Questions

Buprenorphine is frequently used for the treatment of prescription opioid addiction, but the research supporting this has not been fully developed. We do not know who are the best candidates for buprenorphine therapy, or who should be provided an abstinence-based approach. We do not know the optimal duration of treatment, and long-term studies are lacking. Also, we lack good information about the problems with detoxification after long-term maintenance treatment and about what happens after use of buprenorphine. Some of my colleagues give buprenorphine to all the opioid addicts they see; others do not give it to any opioid addicts. The extremes are not unusual in the addiction field, so it is necessary for researchers to provide the information that can set a standard and provide clinicians with good decision-making tools. The clients described in maintenance studies are quite different from those using heroin; they are younger, with less intravenous use, fewer medical consequences, and they are more compliant with treatment expectations (Moore et al. 2007). Perhaps prescription opioid addicts need less treatment with maintenance medications than do heroin addicts and more programs using an abstinence approach. There is a high dropout rate in maintenance treatment within the first year, and a high rate of other substance use. These factors suggest outcomes that are in many ways no different from abstinence approaches; in fact, they could be less effective. We just don't know.

A Reasonable Approach

Buprenorphine is a good medication for opioid detoxification. It tends to work better than the alternatives and provides a relatively smooth transition into a drug-free state. It is certainly preferred by opioid addicts. It makes sense to use abstinence-based approaches for those with prescription opioid addiction that is not severe or long lasting. I have difficulty with colleagues who place people on long-term maintenance therapy (perhaps years) after short-term (six months) prescription opioid dependence. If use has been under a year or two, I do not usually recommend maintenance treatment unless other factors are paramount, like an unstable living situation, poor recovery support, long-term addiction to other substances, and significant co-occurring psychiatric illness. I recommend use of maintenance buprenorphine for many prescription opioid addicts who have had high-dose use of at least a year or two, and I prefer to discuss a definite end point for the maintenance treatment, perhaps nine to eighteen months. If people have been using intravenously or smoking opioids regularly, I am more likely to suggest maintenance therapy. This recommendation takes into account ongoing involvement in psychosocial treatments and recovery activities, such as Twelve Step programs. I believe there is a small population of prescription opioid addicts who need long-term and even lifelong maintenance treatment, but the research has not been done and predictors are unavailable to us, so I do not know who these people are. Those opioid addicts who use a maintenance therapy and become actively involved in long-term treatment and Twelve Step programs should be considered for detoxification and abstinence-based treatment.

Naltrexone

Naltrexone is a mu-opioid antagonist; it blocks the effects of opioids, including intoxication. It has been described as the perfect medication for opioid addiction, because it specifically blocks the reinforcing properties of opioids—people don't get high if they use opioids while taking naltrexone. Unfortunately, most people don't stay with this therapy. They frequently stop taking it and return to opioid use.

Description

Naltrexone is approved by the FDA for treatment of opioid dependence. Only the oral formulation is approved for this use. Thus, an opioid addict must take a naltrexone tablet daily to gain the benefits of the medication. Naltrexone is also approved for the treatment of alcoholism, in two formulations: oral and intramuscular, which is a depot formulation that lasts a month. This depot formulation is being studied for opioid addiction and will most likely be approved for this use soon. Most people find it easier to receive an injection once a month than to take a pill daily. Improved compliance should result in better outcomes. Depot naltrexone is already being used regularly among health care professionals with opioid addiction and the results are very promising (Washington Physicians Health Program 2010).

Pros

The use of naltrexone in the general opioid addict population has not been successful, but it has worked out well for physicians and business executives (Washton, Gold, and Pottash 1984). Monitored use of naltrexone is the norm for the ongoing treatment of physicians with an opioid addiction. It helps to maintain abstinence (Washington Physicians Health Program 2010). Naltrexone has few side effects and is well tolerated by most people. It appears that the depot formulation has resulted in positive outcomes (Comer and Collins 2002; Comer et al. 2006), which supports further research that has not yet been published.

Cons

The poor retention rates of opioid addicts in treatment with naltrexone have resulted in diminished use of this medication for opioid addiction. A Cochrane meta-analysis revealed the disappointing data (Minozzi et al. 2006). It is not widely used for the treatment of opioid addiction due to these poor outcomes. Craving does continue while people take naltrexone compared to reduced craving with maintenance therapies. Patients must wait five to ten days after their last opioid use before initiating naltrexone, or the individual could go into opioid withdrawal. This is a long time for people who have just stopped opioids and are experiencing cravings.

Side Effects

Nausea is the most common side effect of naltrexone use. Less than 10% of those who use it also experience headache, dizziness, anxiety, fatigue, insomnia, vomiting, and drowsiness. On a rare occasion patients using naltrexone feel "dull or numb," or lack their usual joy in life. It can rarely cause liver toxicity, which must be monitored. The primary risk is that of precipitating opioid withdrawal by providing it too soon after the last use of an opioid.

Unanswered Questions

It has been shown that those with high motivation and with a high level of monitoring do well on naltrexone (Washton, Gold, and Pottash 1984). It will be interesting to see if compliance and positive outcomes improve significantly enough with depot naltrexone to result in renewed interest in this treatment of opioid addiction. It is unclear how long one needs to take this medication. Studies have not compared naltrexone treatment to buprenorphine or methadone maintenance, but this would be worthy of attention to help guide clinical decision making.

A Reasonable Approach

Naltrexone is effective in reducing opioid use when it is provided in highly monitored settings. As a result, it can be used with health care professionals in most states or by those who have the money or access to set up such systems. Although a significant level of structure and monitoring is required to ensure compliance with the medication, some clinics and pharmacies could arrange for this. I would suggest use of the depot formulation, off label, for some opioid addicts who cannot or will not consider maintenance treatments, as it has been effective with health care professionals and business executives (Washton, Gold, and Pottash 1984).

Abstinence-based Twelve Step Programs

Abstinence-based Twelve Step programs are treating prescription opioid addicts with a model that requires detoxification and complete abstinence. This model is the prevalent residential treatment model in the United States and is commonly used in outpatient addiction treatment as well. In general, the proponents of this model are unsupportive of maintenance treatment of opioid addiction. They often argue that the individual on maintenance is still taking an addictive substance.

Description

The abstinence-based model of treatment was established by Hazelden in 1949. It requires abstinence from all addicting substances and involvement in Twelve Step programs to support ongoing recovery. This model uses a multidisciplinary team to provide a holistic treatment experience. The primary goals are abstinence from all addicting substances and elimination of addictive behavior, not just abstinence from a class of drugs. Some people would say the long-term goal is life transformation, such that the addict has changed to the point that drug use is no longer needed. The treatment consists of therapy, education, and fellowship. The model uses the Twelve Step philosophy of Alcoholics Anonymous (AA) as a foundation for therapeutic change (Stinchfield and Owen 1998). Psychotherapy is primarily done in a group setting, but individual therapies are also provided. Education about addiction and skills training to promote recovery behaviors helps to inform people about their disease and provide the means of addressing it. Fellowship is found in the strength and support addicts gain from one another as they face a common problem. Co-occurring psychiatric and medical illness is addressed with addiction in an integrated manner.

Pros

The research of this model is limited but reveals very positive outcomes: 53% total abstinence at one year (Stinchfield and Owen 1998). This number is quite similar for alcohol and heroin. The research specific to prescribed opioids is not published, but Hazelden's Butler Center for Research maintains an internal database that reveals 52% total abstinence at one year. Residential treatment provides a setting to get away from the triggers and cues that can result in relapse and provides a period of social, physical, and psychological stabilization. It is also ideal for those with significant co-occurring psychiatric and medical illness, which can be stabilized in such a setting. Another advantage of this model is the emphasis on recovery as a lifestyle, not an event. People are encouraged to attend Twelve Step groups, and to do so for life. They receive a great deal of support at virtually no cost in Twelve Step programs. They gain social support with a group of people who understand addiction and no longer use drugs or alcohol. The cost of residential addiction treatment is high, but the cost of outpatient treatment is low and the cost of ongoing involvement in a Twelve Step program is negligible—people can donate a dollar or two a meeting but are not required to do so. Twelve Step programs are accessible and readily available.

Cons

Residential treatment is very expensive and requires a distinct period of time away from home, family, and work. It lasts from thirty days to several months. This model requires an ongoing effort, although that can be said for all forms of treatment for any chronic disease. There is a marked variation among the different treatment programs and among the counselors, so it can be difficult to find high-quality care. Naltrexone would be acceptable for use in most of the abstinence-based Twelve Step programs, but in general they do not support use of maintenance medications. This is changing to a slight degree within some programs that provide their basic therapies while maintaining people on buprenorphine. The long-term goal is always total abstinence, so people would be asked to engage in recovery activities and at some point they would be advised to discontinue maintenance therapy. Hazelden is providing such treatment at its Florida facility.

Side Effects

The potential for relapse exists with every form of treatment for opioid addiction. People with a history of intravenous drug use, especially heroin use, and who are not on a maintenance therapy may be more likely to relapse and put themselves back at risk for HIV and hepatitis C. This is not necessarily true for users of prescription opioids and the data from buprenorphine and methadone maintenance are not convincing that someone with the time and means to enter into high-quality treatment using an abstinence-based Twelve Step model is at any higher risk of relapse and these significant medical consequences.

Unanswered Questions

Is this form of treatment as effective, more effective, or less effective than the maintenance therapies? This is unknown; however, for inner-city heroin addicts, I would readily endorse use of maintenance therapies based on the research. We do not have a clear understanding of the appropriate length of treatment or who is best suited to an abstinence-based approach. We could benefit from research using a combination of this approach with buprenorphine maintenance to determine whether it was more effective over the long run, if people were able to discontinue buprenorphine and remain active in Twelve Step programs, and how long they needed to be on maintenance therapy.

A Reasonable Approach

The abstinence-based Twelve Step model should be considered for all prescription opioid addicts. Perhaps it should be tried prior to use of maintenance therapies for all but those with severe, intravenous opioid addiction. I suggest use of high-quality programs with a proven track record that use this model along with evidence-based practices. It is of great benefit to have outcome data to use in making such a decision, but it is not published by most of these programs. Long-term involvement in Twelve Step programs is essential to ongoing abstinence and must be emphasized.

Combination Therapy

The use of maintenance therapy within the context of an abstinence-based

Twelve Step program is well known to me from an outpatient program I developed for a treatment center in Portland, Oregon. This experience is informing Hazelden's plans to do the same in its Florida facility. Unfortunately, in Portland we did not do research to inform our decision-making or to define our outcomes, but I will describe it here to provide an understanding of how such a program can work.

Description

We established a standard abstinence-based Twelve Step outpatient addiction treatment program in Portland that met three times a week for two months, twice a week for two months, followed by once a week. Patients were expected to attend treatment group therapy, meet with their counselor individually once a week, and attend Twelve Step meetings a couple times a week. Patients with opioid addiction were evaluated for maintenance therapy and outpatient treatment, or for detoxification and outpatient treatment. They were placed into group therapy with addicts of all kinds: alcoholics, methamphetamine addicts, and marijuana addicts. The counselors were accepting of maintenance treatment, especially after some experience witnessing how it allowed certain opioid addicts to engage in the treatment process who otherwise would not have done so. We consistently described a distinct period of buprenorphine use, nine to eighteen months, with plans to ultimately taper and detoxify people so they could discontinue buprenorphine once a stable period of recovery was established. We provided standard buprenorphine maintenance therapy but required that people attend outpatient treatment to remain in the maintenance program. They could leave the program for other buprenorphine maintenance providers if they chose to, but this was rare.

Experience

The program was readily accepted by patients and their families. The model was effective in that we used two powerful tools to address opioid addiction. Although most of our opioid-addicted patients were using prescription opioids, some used heroin. We had basically two age groups: a group in their late teens through late twenties who began using opioids after experimentation with other drugs, and a group of people in their forties and fifties who for the most part had previously abused other substances but who had also experienced pain, necessitating use of opioids.

The group therapy worked out very well, even with detoxified opioid-addicted patients combined with those on maintenance. They regularly compared notes and we discussed the decision making that separated them into these two treatment models as due to medical decisions to alleviate comparisons. Rarely we detoxified someone from opioids and later started maintenance treatment, but it was always considered an option if people felt they were having significant craving or were at risk for relapse. The two groups were consistently comparing themselves, with the maintenance group doing better early on as they were stabilized on buprenorphine. The abstinent group tended to have an easier time later in treatment, as they had already gone through detoxification, which often scared the buprenorphine group. The buprenorphine group described side effects that made the other group glad to be drug free as well.

Our experience was extremely positive. We had success in both groups and very good treatment retention. The buprenorphine group usually began to seek discontinuation before we suggested it. However, that was not always true—some were so afraid of stopping opioids altogether that it became a real struggle prior to the actual event. I was a poor predictor of those who would benefit from longer-term maintenance therapy. One woman with significant chronic pain chose to discontinue buprenorphine long before I thought it was prudent. A young heroin addict decided to discontinue buprenorphine after several months, which I advised against. He had a one-night relapse to heroin, immediately called and got back on a very low dose of buprenorphine, 2 mg, with complete relief of craving. After a few more months, he successfully discontinued the medication and remained very active in NA.

Most of the group members attended AA, rather than NA meetings; they just felt more comfortable with AA. They did have some minor problems describing their use of buprenorphine and occasionally had to change meetings to find accepting groups, but if they told AA members about it, they described it as a medical treatment necessary for a period of time.

I was glad to have people doing two things to promote abstinence from opioids. I had the opportunity to support their recovery with and without medications. My experience convinced me that individual decision making is essential and that these two models can work very well in an integrated manner. If we are open to the needs of those who seek our expertise, listen to what they want, provide the best information available to them about treatment options in a manner that emphasizes their best chance for positive outcomes, and monitor progress with an open mind for alternative decisions, we will help people engage in treatment, stay in treatment, and with that they will have better outcomes. I'm hopeful that Hazelden will have a similar experience at its Florida facility, and we can do the studies necessary to prove the efficacy of such a combination model.

Learning from Physicians

Addiction treatment outcome studies have a standard set by physicians in recovery from multiple types of addiction. Physicians have the highest recorded abstinence rates, equaled only by pilots, at between 74% and 90% (McLellan et al. 2008; Dupont et al. 2009; Domino et al. 2005). Physicians also have a high rate of abuse of prescribed opioids, 32% and 35% in two samples (McLellan et al. 2008; Domino et al. 2005). Some of the opioids used, like fentanyl and sufentanil, are used intravenously and are remarkably more powerful than heroin. Sufentanil is five to ten times more potent than fentanyl. Fentanyl is one hundred times more potent than morphine while heroin—the opioid that tends to have a dreaded status in our culture as incredibly addicting and powerful in its pure form (which is seldom found on the street)—is only two to four times more potent than morphine.

Some of these physicians are using medications that are hundreds of times more powerful than heroin, they have the best recovery rates measured, and the method of treatment is the abstinence-based Twelve Step model for 95% of them (McLellan et al. 2008). In this study, 78% attended residential treatment for seventy-two days on average. They receive extensive follow-up and monitoring through their state physician health programs, which includes but is not limited to group therapy, individual therapy, Twelve Step meetings, a monthly monitoring meeting, a drug screening, and a workplace monitor. They have extensive treatment and monitoring as well as extremely good motivation for abstinence; they cannot continue to work as physicians if they do not remain abstinent. Of the 904 physicians studied by McLellan and colleagues, only one used methadone and 46 were prescribed naltrexone for opioids or alcohol dependence (2008). The pharmacotherapies are rarely used. The physicians stay abstinent without the use of the maintenance therapies. This is an unusual group, with means to extensive treatment and follow-up, but this data show that maintenance treatments are not essential to recovery from opioid addiction, even from the most powerful opioids on the planet. It suggests that intravenous opioid addicts have multiple options, not just maintenance therapies.

SUMMARY

We need to take all this information into account as we make decisions about treatment for prescription opioid addiction. Addiction treatment needs to be individualized, based on the best treatment available, using the best information about addiction and the best information about the individual. We do not have all the answers, and it is a new specialty, with many opinions, but the professionals in the field must refrain from dogma and stay open to the many possibilities that exist for the person with this unrelenting illness. We need a great deal more research about treatment models for prescription opioid addiction. As this information is gathered, we will determine better treatment planning for those in need and outcomes will improve. The rapidly advancing toll of prescription opioid addiction requires our best efforts.

REFERENCES

Adams, E. H., S. Breiner, T. J. Cicero, A. Geller, J. A. Inciardi, S. H. Schnoll, E. C. Senay, and G. E. Woody. 2006. A comparison of the abuse liability of tramadol, NSAIDs, and hydrocodone in patients with chronic pain. *Journal of Pain and Symptom Management* 31:465–76.

Adler, J. 2003. In the grip of a deeper pain. *Newsweek,* October 20.

Aitken, C., P. Higgs, and M. Hellard. 2008. Buprenorphine injection in Melbourne, Australia—an update. *Drug and Alcohol Review* 27 (2): 197–99.

Alford, R. 2005. Arrests of elderly rising in prescription drug sales. Associated Press, December 13. Cited in Prescription drug abuse: What is being done to address this new drug epidemic? Testimony before the Subcommittee on Criminal Justice, Drug Policy and Human Resources by L. Manchikanti. *Pain Physician* 9 (2006): 287–321.

American Medical Association (AMA). 1990. *Balancing the response to prescription drug abuse: Report of a national symposium on medicine and public policy.* Chicago: American Medical Association, Department of Substance Abuse. Cited in Addiction: Part II. Identification and management of the drug-seeking patient by L. P. Longo, T. Parran, B. Johnson, and W. Kinsey. *American Family Physician* 61 (2000): 2401–8.

American Pain Society. 1995. Treatment of pain at the end of life. Available at: www.ampainsoc.org/advocacy/treatment.htm.

American Psychiatric Association. 2000. *Diagnostic and statistical manual of mental disorders.* 4th ed., text rev. Washington, DC: American Psychiatric Association.

American Society of Addiction Medicine (ASAM). 2009. *Principles of addiction medicine.* 4th ed. Eds. R. Ries, D. Fiellin, S. Miller, and R. Saitz. Philadelphia: Lippincott Williams and Wilkins.

Anglin, M. Douglas. 1998. The natural history of opiate addiction. In *NIH Consensus Development Conference on Effective Medical Treatment of Heroin Addiction.* Available at: www.nih.gov.

Anonymous. 1881. The opium habit. *Catholic World* 33 (September):828. Cited in *The American disease: Origins of narcotic control.* 3rd ed. by D. F. Musto. New York: Oxford University Press, 1999.

Aquina, C. T., A. Marques-Baptista, P. Bridgeman, and M. A. Merlin. 2009. OxyContin abuse and overdose. *Postgraduate Medicine* 121 (2): 163–67.

Argoff, C. E., and D. I. Silvershein. 2009. A comparison of long- and short-acting opioids for the treatment of chronic noncancer pain: Tailoring therapy to meet patient needs. *Mayo Clinic Proceedings* 84 (7): 602–12.

Armstrong, S. C., and K. L. Cozza. 2003. Pharmacokinetic drug interactions of morphine, codeine, and their derivatives: Theory and clinical reality, part II. *Psychosomatics* 44:515–20.

Arria, A. M., K. M. Caldeira, K. B. Vincent, K. E. O'Grady, and E. D. Wish. 2008. Perceived harmfulness predicts nonmedical use of prescription drugs among college students: Interactions with sensation-seeking. *Prevention Science* 9 (3): 191–201.

Associated Press. 2007. Drugmaker to pay $19.5 million to settle OxyContin lawsuit. May 9.

Aston-Jones, G., and G. C. Harris. 2004. Brain substrates for increased drug seeking during protracted withdrawal. *Neuropharmacology* 47 (Suppl 1): 167–79.

Baker, D. E. 2007. Loperamide: A pharmacological review. *Reviews in Gastroenterological Disorders* 7 (Suppl 3): S11–18.

Ball, J. C., and A. Ross. 1991. *The effectiveness of methadone maintenance treatment.* New York: Springer-Verlag, 283.

Batiste, C. G., and L. Yablonsky. 1971. Synanon: A therapeutic life style. *Western Journal of Medicine* 114:90–95.

Bause, G. S. 2009. Sertürner crystallizes morphine. *Anesthesiology* 111 (6): 1307.

Berridge, V., and G. Edwards. 1981. *Opium and the people: Opiate use in nineteenth-century England.* New York: St. Martin's. Cited in *The American disease: Origins of narcotic control.* 3rd ed. by D. F. Musto. New York: Oxford University Press, 1999.

———. 1987. *Opium and the people.* New Haven, CT: Yale University Press.

Bickel, W. K., and L. Amass. 1995. Buprenorphine treatment of opioid dependence: A review. *Experimental and Clinical Psychopharmacology* 3:477–89.

Bieber, C. M., K. Fernandez, D. Borsook, M. J. Brennan, S. F. Butler, R. N. Jamison, E. Osgood, J. Sharpe-Potter, H. N. Thomson, R. D. Weiss, and N. P. Katz. 2008. Retrospective accounts of initial subjective effects of opioids in patients treated for pain who do or do not develop opioid addiction: A pilot case-control study. *Experimental and Clinical Psychopharmacology* 16 (5): 429–34.

Birnbaum, H. G., A. G. White, J. L. Reynolds, P. E. Greenberg, M. Zhang, S. Vallow, J. R. Schein, and N. P. Katz. 2006. Estimated costs of prescription opioid analgesic abuse in the United States in 2001: A societal perspective. *Clinical Journal of Pain* 22 (8): 667–76.

Bishop, E. S. 1919. Narcotic drug addiction: A public health problem. *American Journal of Public Health* 7:481–89.

Black, J. R. 1889. Advantages of substituting the morphia habit for the incurably alcoholic, Cincinnati Lancet-Clinic. Cited in *Opiate addiction* by A. R. Lindesmith, Evanston, IL: Principia Press, 1947: 183. Cited in *Licit and illicit drugs: The consumers union report on narcotics, stimulants, depressants, inhalants, hallucinogens, and marijuana—including caffeine, nicotine, and alcohol* by E. M. Brecher and the editors of *Consumer Reports.* Boston: Little, Brown and Company, 1972.

Blair Historic Preservation Alliance. Available at: www.blairhistory.com/archive/keeley_cure/default.htm.

Booth, M. 1996. *Opium: A history.* London: Simon and Schuster.

Boyd, C. J., S. E. McCabe, J. A. Cranford, and A. Young. 2006. Adolescents' motivations to abuse prescription medications. *Pediatrics* 118 (6): 2472–80.

Boyer, E. W., M. Shannon, and P. L. Hibberd. 2005. The Internet and psychoactive substance use among innovative drug users. *Pediatrics* 115:302–5.

Boyes, J. H. 1931. Medical history: Dover's powder and Robinson Crusoe. *New England Journal of Medicine* 204:440–43. Cited in *Licit and illicit drugs: The consumers union report on narcotics, stimulants, depressants, inhalants, hallucinogens, and marijuana—including caffeine, nicotine, and alcohol* by E. M. Brecher and the editors of *Consumer Reports.* Boston: Little, Brown and Company, 1972.

Brecher, E. M., and the editors of *Consumer Reports.* 1972. *Licit and illicit drugs: The consumers union report on narcotics, stimulants, depressants, inhalants, hallucinogens, and marijuana—including caffeine, nicotine, and alcohol.* Boston: Little, Brown and Company.

Breiter, H. C., R. L. Gollub, R. M. Weisskoff, D. N. Kennedy, N. Makris, J. D. Berke, J. M. Goodman, H. L. Kantor, D. R. Gastfriend, J. P. Riorden, R. T. Mathew, B. R. Rosen, S. E. Hyman. 1997. Acute effects of cocaine on human brain activity and emotion. *Neuron* 19 (3): 591–611.

Brookoff, D. 1993. Abuse potential of various opioid medications. *Journal of General Internal Medicine* 8:688–90.

Brotman, R., and A. M. Freedman. 1968. *A community mental health approach to drug addiction.* Washington, DC: U.S. Department of Health, Education, and Welfare.

Brownstein, J. S., T. C. Green, T. A. Cassidy, and S. F. Butler. 2010. Geographic information systems and pharmacoepidemiology: Using spatial cluster detection to monitor local patterns of prescription opioid abuse. *Pharmacoepidemiology and Drug Safety* 19:627–37.

Budman, S. H., J. M. G. Serrano, and S. F. Butler. 2009. Can abuse deterrent formulations make a difference? Expectation and speculation. *Harm Reduction Journal* 6:8–15.

Butler, S. F., S. H. Budman, K. C. Fernandez, B. Houle, C. Benoit, N. Katz, and R. N. Jamison. 2007. Development and validation of the Current Opioid Misuse Measure. *Pain* 130 (1–2): 144–56.

Butler, S. F., K. Fernandez, C. Benoit, S. H. Budman, and R. N. Jamison. 2008. Validation of the Revised Screener and Opioid Assessment for Patients with Pain (SOAPP-R). *Journal of Pain* 9 (4): 360–72.

Califano, J. A. 2007. High society: How substance abuse ravages America and what to do about it. New York: Perseus Publishing. Cited in National drug control policy and prescription drug abuse: Facts and fallacies by L. Manchikanti. *Pain Physician* 10:399–424.

Casey, E. 1978. History of drug use and drug users in the United States. In *Facts about drug abuse: Participant manual.* The National Drug Abuse Center for Training Resource and Development. Publication No. 79-FADA-041P, November. Available at: www.druglibrary.org/schaffer/History/CASEY1.htm.

Caywood, T. 2003. Online drug buying can turn into a nasty habit: Deals are illegal, dangerous, *Boston Herald,* December 14. Cited in Prescription drug abuse: What is being done to address this new drug epidemic? Testimony before the Subcommittee on Criminal Justice, Drug Policy and Human Resources by L. Manchikanti. *Pain Physician* 9 (2006): 287–321.

Center for Substance Abuse Treatment (CSAT). 2004a. *Clinical guidelines for the use of buprenorphine in the treatment of opioid addiction.* Treatment Improvement Protocol (TIP) Series 40. DHHS Publication No. (SMA) 04-3939. Rockville, MD: Substance Abuse and Mental Health Services Administration.

———. 2004b. Methadone-Associated Mortality: Report of a National Assessment, May 8–9, 2003. CSAT Publication No. 28-03. Rockville, MD: Substance Abuse and Mental Health Services Administration. Cited in Prescription drug abuse: What is being done to address this new drug epidemic? Testimony before the Subcommittee on Criminal Justice, Drug Policy and Human Resources by L. Manchikanti. *Pain Physician* 9 (2006): 287–321.

———. 2008. OxyContin: Prescription drug abuse—2008 revision. *Substance Abuse Treatment Advisory* vol. 7, issue 1. Rockville, MD: Substance Abuse and Mental Health Services Administration. Available at: www.samhsa.gov.

Chappel, J. N., and R. L. DuPont. 1999. Twelve-step and mutual-help programs for addictive disorders. *Psychiatric Clinics of North America* 22:425–46.

Chrisman, C. R. 2003. Protease inhibitor-drug interactions: Proceed with caution. *Journal of Critical Illness* 18 (4): 185–88.

Christo, G., and C. Franey. 1995. Drug users' spiritual beliefs, locus of control and the disease concept in relation to Narcotics Anonymous attendance and six-month outcomes. *Drug and Alcohol Dependence* 38:51–56.

Christo, G., and S. Sutton. 1994. Anxiety and self-esteem as a function of abstinence time among recovering addicts attending Narcotics Anonymous. *British Journal of Clinical Psychology* 33:198–200.

Chua, S. M., and T. S. Lee. 2006. Abuse of prescription buprenorphine, regulatory controls and the role of the primary physician. *Annals of the Academy of Medicine, Singapore* 35:492–95.

Cicero, T. J., C. N. Shores, A. G. Paradis, and M. S. Ellis. 2008. Source of drugs for prescription opioid analgesic abusers: A role for the Internet? *Pain Medicine* 9 (6): 718–23.

Cicero T., H. Surratt, and J. Inciardi. 2007. Use and misuse of buprenorphine in the management of opioid addiction. *Journal of Opioid Management* 3 (6): 302–8.

Clark, N. H. 1976. *Deliver us from evil: An interpretation of American prohibition.* New York: W.W. Norton. Cited in *Licit and illicit drugs: The consumers union report on narcotics, stimulants, depressants, inhalants, hallucinogens, and marijuana—including caffeine, nicotine, and alcohol* by E. M. Brecher and the editors of *Consumer Reports.* Boston: Little, Brown and Company, 1972.

Clines, F. X., and B. Meier. 2001. Cancer painkillers pose new abuse threat. *New York Times,* February 9.

Colameco, S., J. S. Coren, and C. A. Ciervo. 2009. Continuous opioid treatment for chronic noncancer pain: A time for moderation in prescribing. *Postgraduate Medicine* 121 (4): 61–66.

Cole, N. 2004. Rx roulette on the Internet. *Wall Street Journal,* June 17: A18. Cited in Prescription drug abuse: What is being done to address this new drug epidemic? Testimony before the Subcommittee on Criminal Justice, Drug Policy and Human Resources by L. Manchikanti. *Pain Physician* 9 (2006): 287–321.

Columbia Daily Tribune. 2002. Health-care worker drug abuse rising, statistics suggest. Available at: http://archive.showmenews.com/2002/Mar/20020330News015.asp (Accessed on April 6, 2005). Cited in Ephemeral profiles of prescription drug and formulation tampering: Evolving pseudoscience on the Internet by E. J. Cone. *Drug and Alcohol Dependence* 83 (2006): S31–39.

Comer, S. D., and E. D. Collins. 2002. Depot naltrexone: Long-lasting antagonism of the effects of heroin in humans. *Psychopharmacology* 159 (4): 351–60.

Comer, S. D., M. A. Sullivan, E. Yu, J. L. Rothenberg, H. D. Kleber, K. Kampman, C. Dackis, and C. P. O'Brien. 2006. Injectable, sustained-release naltrexone for the treatment of opioid dependence: A randomized, placebo-controlled trial. *Archives of General Psychiatry* 63 (2): 210–18.

Compton, W. M., and N. D. Volkow. 2006. Major increases in opioid analgesic abuse in the United States: Concerns and strategies. *Drug and Alcohol Dependence* 81 (2): 103–7.

Cone, E. J. 2006. Ephemeral profiles of prescription drug and formulation tampering: Evolving pseudoscience on the Internet. *Drug and Alcohol Dependence* 83 (Suppl 1): S31–39.

Cone, E. J., H. A. Heit, Y. H. Caplan, and D. Gourlay. 2006. Evidence of morphine metabolism to hydromorphone in pain patients chronically treated with morphine. *Journal of Analytical Toxicology* 30:1–5.

Conlin, M. F. 1990. States starting to target Rx drugs sold on the streets. *Drug Topics* 6:44.

Cooper, J. R., F. Altman, B. S. Brown, and D. Czechowicz. 1983. *Research on the treatment of narcotic addiction: State of the art.* Rockville, MD: National Institute on Drug Abuse.

Cooper, O. B., T. T. Brown, and A. S. Dobs. 2003. Opiate drug use: A potential contributor to the endocrine and metabolic complications in human immunodeficiency virus disease. *Clinical Infectious Diseases* 37 (Suppl 2): S132–36.

Courtwright, D. T. 1982. *Dark paradise: Opiate addiction in America before 1940.* Cambridge, MA: Harvard University Press. Cited in Drugs and race in American culture: Orientalism in the turn-of-the-century discourse of narcotic addiction by T. A. Hickman. *American Studies* 41 (2000): 71–91.

———. 1985. *Dark paradise.* Cambridge, MA: Harvard University Press.

———. 1992. A century of American narcotic policy. In D. R. Gerstein and H. J. Harwood, eds. *Treating drug problems.* Vol. 2. Institute of Medicine. Washington, DC: National Academy Press.

———. 2001. *Dark paradise.* Cambridge, MA: Harvard University Press.

———. 2004. The Controlled Substances Act: How a "big tent" reform became a punitive drug law. *Drug and Alcohol Dependence* 76:9–15.

Crape, B. L., C. A. Latkin, A. S. Laris, and A. R. Knowlton. 2002. The effects of sponsorship in Twelve Step treatment of injection drug users. *Drug and Alcohol Dependence* 65:291–301.

Cross, G. M., C. W. Morgan, A. J. Mooney, C. A. Martin, and J. A. Rafter. 1990. Alcoholism treatment: A ten-year follow-up study. *Alcoholism, Clinical and Experimental Research* 14:169–73.

Curtis, L. H., J. Stoddard, J. I. Radeva, S. Hutchison, P. E. Dans, A. Wright, R. L. Woosley, and K. A. Schulman. 2006. Geographic variation in the prescription of schedule II opioid analgesics among outpatients in the United States. *Health Services Research* 41 (3 Pt 1): 837–55.

Daglish, M. R. C., A. Weinstein, A. L. Malizia, S. Wilson, J. K. Melichar, S. Britten, C. Brewer, A. Lingford-Hughes, J. S. Myles, P. Grasby, and D. J. Nutt. 2001. Changes in regional cerebral blood flow elicited by craving memories in abstinent opiate-dependent subjects. *American Journal of Psychiatry* 158:1680–86.

Dahan, A. 2006. Opioid-induced respiratory effects: New data on buprenorphine. *Palliative Medicine* 20 (8): 3–8.

Darke, S., and W. Hall. 2003. Heroin overdose: Research and evidence-based intervention. *Journal of Urban Health* 80:189–200.

Dasgupta, N., F. M. Jonsson, and J. S. Brownstein. 2008. Comparing unintentional opioid poisoning mortality in metropolitan and non-metropolitan counties, United States, 1999–2003. In *Geography and Drug Addiction,* edited by Y. Thomas, D. Richardson, and I. Cheung. Berlin: Springer Publishers. Cited in Can abuse deterrent formulations make a difference? Expectation and speculation by S. H. Budman, J. M. G. Serrano, and S. F. Butler. *Harm Reduction Journal* 6 (2009): 8–15.

Davids, E., and M. Gastpar. 2004. Buprenorphine in the treatment of opioid dependence. *European Neuropsychopharmacology* 14:209–16.

Davis, M. P., J. Varga, D. Dickerson, D. Walsh, S. B. LeGrand, and R. Lagman. 2003. Normal-release and controlled-release oxycodone: Pharmacokinetics, pharmacodynamics, and controversy. *Supportive Care in Cancer* 11:84–92.

Davis, W. R., and B. D. Johnson. 2008. Prescription opioid use, misuse, and diversion among street drug users in New York City. *Drug and Alcohol Dependence* January 1; 92 (1–3): 267–76.

Day, H. 1868. *The opium habit.* Cited in *The opium problem* by C. E. Terry and M. Pellens. New York: Committee on Drug Addictions, Bureau of Social Hygiene, 1928: 5. Cited in *Licit and illicit drugs: The consumers union report on narcotics, stimulants, depressants, inhalants, hallucinogens, and marijuana—including caffeine, nicotine, and alcohol* by E. M. Brecher and the editors of *Consumer Reports.* Boston: Little, Brown and Company, 1972.

Denisco, R. A., R. K. Chandler, and W. M. Compton. 2008. Addressing the intersecting problems of opioid misuse and chronic pain treatment. *Experimental and Clinical Psychopharmacology* 16 (5): 417–28.

deWit, H., B. Bodker, and J. Ambre. 1992. Rate of increase of plasma drug level influences subjective response in humans. *Psychopharmacology* 107:352–58.

deWit, H., S. Dudish, and J. Ambre. 1993. Subjective and behavioral effects of diazepam depend on its rate of onset. *Psychopharmacology* 112:324–30.

Dole, V. P. 1970. Biochemistry of addiction. *Annual Review of Biochemistry* 39:821–40.

———. 1972. Narcotic addiction, physical dependence and relapse. *New England Journal of Medicine* 286:988–92.

———. 1988. Implications of methadone maintenance for theories of narcotic addiction. *JAMA* 260 (20): 3025–29.

———. 1991. Addiction as a public health problem. *Alcoholism, Clinical and Experimental Research* 15 (5): 749–52.

———. 1994. Methadone maintenance: Optimizing dosage by estimating plasma level. *Journal of Addictive Diseases* 12:1–4.

Dole, V. P., and M. E. Nyswander. 1965. A medical treatment for diacetylmorphine (heroin) addiction. *JAMA* 193:80–84.

———. 1967. Heroin addiction: A metabolic disease. *Archives of Internal Medicine* 120:19–24.

Domino, K. B., T. F. Hornbein, N. L. Polissar, G. Renner, J. Johnson, S. Alberti, and L. Hankes. 2005. Risk factors for relapse in health care professionals with substance use disorders. *JAMA* 293 (12): 1453–60.

Drucker, E. 2000. From morphine to methadone: Maintenance drugs in the treatment of opiate addiction. In *Harm reduction: National and international perspectives* edited by J. A. Inciardi and L. D. Harrison. Thousand Oaks, CA: Sage Publications.

Drug Enforcement Administration (DEA). 2004. *Drugs and chemicals of concern: Fentanyl.* Available at: www.deadiversion.usdoj.gov/drugs_concern/fentanyl.htm (Accessed on April 5, 2005). Cited in Ephemeral profiles of prescription drug and formulation tampering: Evolving pseudoscience on the Internet by E. J. Cone. *Drug and Alcohol Dependence* 83 (2006): S31–39.

———. 2005. *Drugs of abuse.* U.S. Department of Justice. Available at: www.justice.gov/dea/pubs/abuse.

Drug Enforcement Administration and the National Alliance for Model State Drug Laws. 2006. *A closer look at state prescription monitoring programs* (www.deadiversion.usdoj.gov/pubs/program/prescription-monitor/summary.htm). Cited in Prescription drug abuse: What is being done to address this new drug epidemic? Testimony before the Subcommittee on Criminal Justice, Drug Policy and Human Resources by L. Manchikanti. *Pain Physician* 9 (2006): 287–321.

Dupont, R. L., A. T. McLellan, W. L. White, L. J. Merlo, and M. S. Gold. 2009. Setting the standard for recovery: Physicians health programs. *Journal of Substance Abuse Treatment* 36:159–71.

Eap, C. B., T. Buclin, and P. Baumann. 2002. Interindividual variability of the clinical pharmacokinetics of methadone: Implications for the treatment of opioid dependence. *Clinical Pharmacokinetics* 41 (14): 1153–93.

Edlund, M. J., M. Sullivan, D. Steffick, K. M. Harris, and K. B. Wells. 2007. Do users of regularly prescribed opioids have higher rates of substance use problems than nonusers? *Pain Medicine* 8 (8): 647–56.

Eriksen, J., P. Sjøgren, E. Bruera, O. Ekholm, and N. K. Rasmussen. 2006. Critical issues on opioids in chronic non-cancer pain: An epidemiological study. *Pain* 125 (1–2): 172–79.

Falco, M. 2006. Testimony of Mathea Falco, president, Drug Strategies, before the Subcommittee on Criminal Justice, Drug Policy and Human Resources, July 26. Cited in Prescription drug abuse: What is being done to address this new drug epidemic? Testimony before the Subcommittee on Criminal Justice, Drug Policy and Human Resources by L. Manchikanti. *Pain Physician* 9 (2006): 287–321.

Farre, M., and J. Cami. 1991. Pharmacokinetic considerations in abuse liability evaluation. *British Journal of Addiction* 86:1601–6.

Fiellin, D. A., G. H. Friedland, and M. N. Gourevitch. 2006. Opioid dependence: Rationale for and efficacy of existing and new treatments. *Clinical Infectious Diseases* 43 (Suppl 4): S173–77.

Finn, P., and K. Wilcock. 1997. Levo-alpha acetyl methadol (LAAM): Its advantages and drawbacks. *Journal of Substance Abuse Treatment* 14:559–64.

Fischer, B., J. Patra, M. F. Cruz, J. Gittins, and J. Rehm. 2008. Comparing heroin users and prescription opioid users in a Canadian multi-site population of illicit opioid users. *Drug and Alcohol Review* 27 (6): 625–32.

Fishbain, D. A., B. Cole, J. Lewis, H. L. Rosomoff, and R. S. Rosomoff. 2008. What percentage of chronic nonmalignant pain patients exposed to chronic opioid analgesic therapy develop abuse/addiction and/or aberrant drug-related behaviors? A structured evidence-based review. *Pain Medicine* 9 (4): 444–59.

Flannagan, L. M., J. D. Butts, and W. H. Anderson. 1996. Fentanyl patches left on dead bodies—potential source of drug for abusers. *Journal of Forensic Sciences* 41:320–21.

Food and Drug Administration (FDA). 2005. FDA asks Purdue Pharma to withdraw Palladone for safety [press release]. July 13. Available at: www.fda.gov/bbs/topics/NEWS/2005/NEW01205.html.

Forman, R. F., D. B. Marlowe, and A. T. McLellan. 2006. The Internet as a source of drugs of abuse. *Current Psychiatry Reports* 8 (5): 377–82.

Frykholm, B. 1985. The drug career. *Journal of Drug Issues* 15:333–46.

Garrido, M. J., and I. F. Troconiz. 1999. Methadone: A review of its pharmacokinetic/pharmacodynamic properties. *Journal of Pharmacological and Toxicological Methods* 42:61–66.

Gerber, J. G. 2002. Interactions between methadone and antiretroviral medications. Paper presented at 3rd International Workshop on Clinical Pharmacology of HIV Therapy [NIDA-sponsored]. April 13; Washington, DC. Cited in Methadone-drug interactions. 3rd ed. by S. B. Leavitt. *Addiction Treatment Forum* (2005). Available at: www.atforum.com/SiteRoot/pages/rxmethadone/methadonedruginteractions.shtml.

Gerstein, D. R., and H. J. Harwood, eds. 1990. *Treating drug problems.* Vol. 1. Institute of Medicine. Washington, DC: National Academy Press.

Gilman, S. M., M. Galanter, and H. Dermatis. 2001. Methadone Anonymous: A Twelve Step program for methadone maintained heroin addicts. *Substance Abuse* 22:247–56.

Glickman, L., M. Galanter, H. Dermatis, and S. Dingle. 2006. Recovery and spiritual transformation among peer leaders of a modified Methadone Anonymous group. *Journal of Psychoactive Drugs* 38:531–33.

Gordon, S. M., R. F. Forman, and C. Siatkowski. 2006. Knowledge and use of the Internet as a source of controlled substances. *Journal of Substance Abuse Treatment* 30:271–74.

Gourevitch, M. N. 2001. Interactions between HIV-related medications and methadone: An overview. (Updated March 2001.) *Mt Sinai Journal of Medicine* 68(3): 227–28.

Green, T. C., and S. F. Butler. 2008. A latent class analysis of prescription opioid abuse in the National Addictions Vigilance Intervention and Prevention Program. Oral presentation at the 70th annual meeting of the College on Problems of Drug Dependence in San Juan, Puerto Rico (June).

Green, T. C., J. M. Grimes Serrano, A. Licari, S. H. Budman, and S. F. Butler. 2009. Women who abuse prescription opioids: Findings from the Addiction Severity Index–Multimedia Version Connect prescription opioid database. *Drug and Alcohol Dependence* 103 (1–2): 65–73.

Gutstein, H. B., and H. Akil. 2006. Opioid analgesics. In *Goodman and Gilman's The Pharmacological Basis of Therapeutics,* 11th ed., L. Brunton, ed., New York: McGraw-Hill, 547–90.

Hakansson, A., A. Medvedeo, M. Andersson, and M. Berglund. 2007. Buprenorphine misuse among heroin and amphetamine users in Malmo, Sweden: Purpose of misuse and route of administration. *European Addiction Research* 13 (4): 207–15.

Hall, A. J., J. E. Logan, R. L. Toblin, J. A. Kaplan, J. C. Kraner, D. Bixler, A. E. Crosby, and L. J. Paulozzi. 2008. Patterns of abuse among unintentional pharmaceutical overdose fatalities. *JAMA* 300 (22): 2613–20.

Harris, A. C., and J. C. Gewirtz. 2005. Acute opioid dependence: Characterizing the early adaptations underlying drug withdrawal. *Psychopharmacology* 178:353–66.

Hartel, D., E. E. Schoenbaum, P. A. Selwyn, E. Drucker, W. Wasserman, and G. H. Friedman. 1989. Temporal patterns of cocaine use and AIDS in intravenous drug users in methadone maintenance. 5th International Conference on AIDS, Stockholm, Sweden (June).

Havens, J. R., R. Walker, and C. G. Leukefeld. 2007. Prevalence of opioid analgesic injection among rural nonmedical opioid analgesic users. *Drug and Alcohol Dependence* 87:98–102.

———. 2008. Prescription opioid use in the rural Appalachia: A community-based study. *Journal of Opioid Management* 4 (2): 63–71.

Hawkins, J. D. 1980. Some suggestions for "self-help" approaches with street drug abusers. *Journal of Psychedelic Drugs* 12:131–37. Cited in *The early impact of involvement in Narcotics Anonymous self-help groups: A report from the Role of Self-Help Groups in Drug Treatment Research Project* by J. W. Toumbourou and M. Hamilton. Fitzroy, Australia: Turning Point Alcohol and Drug Centre, 2003.

Hayes, B. D., W. Klein-Schwartz, and S. Doyon. 2008. Toxicity of buprenorphine overdose in children. *Pediatrics* 121 (4): e782.

Henretig, F., C. Vassalluzo, K. Ousterhoudt, E. W. Boyer, and J. Martin. 1998. Rave by net: Gamma-hydroxybutyrate (GHB) toxicity from kits sold to minors via the Internet. *Journal of Toxicology, Clinical Toxicology* 36:503.

Hentoff, N. 1965. The treatment of patients [Profile of Dr. Marie Nyswander]. *New Yorker* 41 (June 26) 45. Cited in *Dark paradise: A history of opiate addiction in America* by D. T. Courtwright. Cambridge, MA: Harvard University Press, 2001.

Hickman, T. A. 2000. Drugs and race in American culture: Orientalism in the turn-of-the-century discourse of narcotic addiction. *American Studies* 41:71–91.

Higgins, S. T. 1997. The influence of alternative reinforcers on cocaine use and abuse: A brief review. *Pharmacology, Biochemistry, and Behavior* 57:419–27.

Himmelsbach, C. K. 1942. Clinical studies of drug addiction: Physical dependence, withdrawal and recovery. *Archives of Internal Medicine* 69:766–72.

Hitt, E. 2009. FDA panel recommends approval of tamper-resistant oxycodone formulation. September 28. Available at: www.medscape.com/viewarticle/709578.

Homsi, J., D. Walsh, and K. A. Nelson. 2001. Important drugs for cough in advanced cancer. *Supportive Care in Cancer* 9:565–74.

Howard-Jones, N. 1971. The origins of hypodermic medication. *Scientific American,* January.

Hser, Y., M. D. Anglin, C. Grella, D. Longshore, and M. Prendergast. Drug treatment careers: A conceptual framework and existing research findings. Unpublished manuscript.

Hser, Y., M. D. Anglin, and K. Powers. 1993. A 24-year follow-up of California narcotics addicts. *Archives of General Psychiatry* 50:577–84.

Huestis, M. A., A. Umbricht, K. L. Preston, and E. J. Cone. 1999. Safety of buprenorphine: Ceiling effect for subjective measures at high intravenous doses. In *Problems of drug dependence 1998: Proceedings of the 60th Annual Scientific Meeting* edited by L. S. Harris. (NIDA Research Monograph 179, NIH Publication No. 99-4395). Rockville, MD: National Institute on Drug Abuse, 62.

Hugdahl, K., A. Berardi, W. L. Thompson, S. M. Kosslyn, R. Macy, D. P. Baker, N. M. Alpert, and J. E. LeDoux. 1995. Brain mechanisms in human classical conditioning: A PET blood flow study. *Neuroreport* 6:1723–28.

Humphreys, K., S. Wing, D. McCarty, J. Chappel, L. Gallant, B. Haberle, A. T. Horvath, L. A. Kaskutas, Y. Kirk, D. Kivlahan, A. Laudet, B. S. McCrady, A. T. McLellan, J. Morgenstern, M. Townsend, and R. Weiss. 2004. Self-help organizations for alcohol and drug problems: Toward evidence-based practice and policy. *Journal of Substance Abuse Treatment* 26:151–58.

Inciardi, J. A., and J. L. Goode. 2003. OxyContin and prescription drug abuse. *Consumers' Research Magazine,* July:17–19.

Inciardi, J. A., H. L. Surratt, T. J. Cicero, and R. A. Beard. 2009. Prescription opioid abuse and diversion in an urban community: The results of an ultrarapid assessment. *Pain Medicine* 10 (3): 537–48.

Inciardi, J. A., H. L. Surratt, S. P. Kurtz, and T. J. Cicero. 2007. Mechanisms of prescription drug diversion among drug-involved club- and street-based populations. *Pain Medicine* 8 (2): 171–83.

Institute of Medicine. 1990. *Treating drug problems.* Washington, DC: National Academy Press.

Inturrisi, C. E. 2002. Clinical pharmacology of opioids for pain. *Clinical Journal of Pain* 18:S1–12.

Isenhart, C. E. 1997. Pretreatment readiness for change in male alcohol dependent subjects: Predictors of one-year follow-up status. *Journal of Studies on Alcohol* 58:351–57.

Ives, T. J., P. R. Chelminski, C. A. Hammett-Stabler, R. M. Malone, J. S. Perhac, N. M. Potisek, B. B. Shilliday, D. A. DeWalt, and M. P. Pignone. 2006. Predictors of opioid misuse in patients with chronic pain: A prospective cohort study. *BMC Health Services Research* 6 (April 4): 46.

Jaffe, J. H. 1975. The maintenance option and the Special Action Office for Drug Abuse Prevention. *Psychiatric Annals* 5:12–42.

Jaffe, J. H., M. Kanzler, and J. Green. 1980. Abuse potential of loperamide. *Clinical Pharmacology and Therapeutics* 28 (6): 812–19.

Jayawant, S. S., and R. Balkrishnan. 2005. The controversy surrounding OxyContin abuse: Issues and solutions. *Therapeutics and Clinical Risk Management* 1:77–82.

JCABA and AMAND. 1961. *Drug addiction: Crime or disease? Interim and final reports of the Joint Committee of the American Bar Association and the American Medical Association on Narcotic Drugs.* Bloomington, IN: Indiana University Press.

Johnson, B. 1998. The mechanism of codependence in the prescription of benzodiazepines to patients with addiction. *Psychiatric Annals* 28 (3): 166–71.

Joseph, H., S. Stancliff, and J. Langrod. 2000. Methadone maintenance treatment (MMT): A review of historical and clinical issues. *Mount Sinai Journal of Medicine* 67:347–65.

Joseph, H., and J. S. Woods. 2006. In the service of patients: The legacy of Dr. Dole. *Heroin Addiction and Related Clinical Problems* 8 (4): 9–28.

Kahan, M., A. Srivastava, L. Wilson, D. Gourlay, and D. Midmer. 2006. Misuse of and dependence on opioids: Study of chronic pain patients. *Canadian Family Physician* 52:1081–87.

Kalb, C. 2001. Playing with painkillers. *Newsweek,* April 9.

Kane, H. H. 1880. The hypodermic injection of morphia: Its history, advantages, and dangers. Based on experience of 360 physicians (New York). Cited in *Licit and illicit drugs: The consumers union report on narcotics, stimulants, depressants, inhalants, hallucinogens, and marijuana—including caffeine, nicotine, and alcohol* by E. M. Brecher and the editors of *Consumer Reports.* Boston: Little, Brown and Company, 1972.

Karch, S. B. 1998. *Drug abuse handbook.* Boca Raton, FL: CRC Press.

Katz, N. 2008. Abuse-deterrent opioid formulations: Are they a pipe dream? *Current Rheumatology Reports* 10:11–18.

Katz, D. A., and L. R. Hays. 2004. Adolescent OxyContin abuse. *Journal of the American Academy of Child and Adolescent Psychiatry* 43 (2): 231–34.

Katz, J. P., and K. M. Sturmann. 1993. Appendicitis associated with loperamide hydrochloride abuse. *Annals of Pharmacotherapy* 27 (3): 369–70.

Kentucky All Schedule Prescription Electronic Reporting (KASPER). 2006. A comprehensive report on Kentucky's prescription monitoring program prepared by the Cabinet for Health and Family Services Office of the Inspector General, Version 1, 3/29/2006. www.chfs.ky.gov/ NR/rdonlyres/2D46AB2E-FAE8-43DC-9CE6 -6BB4B419918F/0/AComprehensiveSummaryofKASPERDraft.pdf. Cited in Prescription drug abuse: What is being done to address this new drug epidemic? Testimony before the Subcommittee on Criminal Justice, Drug Policy and Human Resources by L. Manchikanti. *Pain Physician* 9 (2006): 287–321.

Khajawall, A. M., J. J. Sramek, and G. M. Simpson. 1982. "Loads" alert. *Western Journal of Medicine* 137:166–68.

Kintz, P. 2001. Death involving buprenorphine: A compendium of French cases. *Forensic Science International* 121 (1): 65.

Koob, G. F. 1992. Drugs of abuse: Anatomy, pharmacology and function of reward pathways. *Trends in Pharmacological Science* 13:177–84.

Koob, G. F., and F. E. Bloom. 1988. Cellular and molecular mechanisms of drug dependence. *Science* 242:715–23.

Koob, G. F., and M. LeMoal. 2001. Drug addiction, dysregulation of reward, and allostasis. *Neuropsychopharmacology* 24 (2): 97–129.

Kooyman, M. 1993. *The therapeutic community for addicts.* Amsterdam: Swets and Zeitlinger.

Kosten, T. R. 1990. Current pharmacotherapies for opioid dependence. *Psychopharmacology Bulletin* 26:69–74.

Kosten, T.R., and T. P. George. 2002. The neurobiology of opioid dependence: Implications for treatment. *Science and Practice Perspectives* 1 (1): 13–20.

Kraman, P. 2004. Drug abuse in America: Prescription drug diversion. TrendsAlert. Lexington, KY: The Council of State Governments. (April). www.csg.org. Cited in Prescription drug abuse: What is being done to address this new drug epidemic? Testimony before the Subcommittee on Criminal Justice, Drug Policy and Human Resources by L. Manchikanti. *Pain Physician* 9 (2006): 287–321.

Krantz, M. J., and P. S. Mehler. 2004. Treating opioid dependence. Growing implications for primary care. *Archives of Internal Medicine* 164:277–88.

Kuehn, B. M. 2007. Opioid prescriptions soar: Increase in legitimate use as well as abuse. *JAMA* 297:249–51.

Kuhne, G. 1926. Statement of Gerhard Kuhne, head of the Identification Bureau, New York City Department of Correction. In *Conference on narcotic education: Hearings before the Committee on Education of the House of Representatives. December 16, 1925.* Washington, DC: U.S. Government Printing Office. Cited in *The American disease: Origins of narcotic control,* 3rd. ed. by D. F. Musto. New York: Oxford University Press, 1999.

Lange, W. R. 1990. Safety and side effects of buprenorphine in the clinical management of heroin addiction. *Drug and Alcohol Dependence* 26:19–28.

Langlitz, N., K. Schotte, and T. Bschor. 2001. [Loperamide abuse in anxiety disorder]. *Der Nervenarzt* 72 (7): 562–64.

Laudet, A. B. 2008. The impact of Alcoholics Anonymous on other substance abuse related Twelve Step programs. *Recent Developments in Alcoholism* 18:71–89.

Laudet, A. B., S. Magura, H. S. Vogel, and E. Knight. 2000. Support, mutual aid and recovery from dual diagnosis. *Community Mental Health Journal* 36:457–76.

Laudet, A., and G. Storey. 2006. A comparison of the recovery experience in the U.S. and Australia: Toward identifying "universal" and culture-specific processes. International NIDA Research Forum. Scottsdale, AZ.

Leavitt, S. B. 2009. Opioid antagonists, naloxone and naltrexone: Aids for pain management; Pain treatment topics. March. Available at: www.pain-topics.org.

Leow, K. P., M. T. Smith, J. A. Watt, B. E. Williams, and T. Cramond. 1992. Comparative oxycodone pharmacokinetics in humans after intravenous, oral, and rectal administration. *Therapeutic Drug Monitoring* 14:479–84.

Lessenger, J. E., and S. D. Feinberg. 2008. Abuse of prescription and over-the-counter medications. *Journal of the American Board of Family Medicine* 21:45–54.

Levine, S. M. 1974. *Narcotics and drug abuse.* Cincinnati, OH: The W. H. Anderson Company. 1973; revised 1974. Cited in *Licit and illicit drugs: The consumers union report on narcotics, stimulants, depressants, inhalants, hallucinogens, and marijuana— including caffeine, nicotine, and alcohol* by E. M. Brecher and the editors of *Consumer Reports.* Boston: Little, Brown and Company, 1972.

Libby, R. T. 2005. Treating doctors as drug dealers: The DEA's war on prescription painkillers. Cato Institute. Policy Analysis #545, June 16.

———. 2008. *The criminalization of medicine in America.* Westport, CT: Praeger Publishers.

Lindesmith, A. R. 1965. *The addict and the law.* Bloomington, IN: University Press. Cited in *Dark paradise: A history of opiate addiction in America* by D. T. Courtwright. Cambridge, MA: Harvard University Press, 2001.

Ling, W., C. Charuvastra, J. F. Collins, S. Batki, L. S. Brown Jr, P. Kintaudi, D. R. Wesson, L. McNicholas, D. J. Tusel, U. Malkerneker, J. A. Renner Jr, E. Santos, P. Casadonte, C. Fye, S. Stine, R. I. Wang, and D. Segal. 1998. Buprenorphine maintenance treatment of opiate dependence: A multicenter, randomized clinical trial. *Addiction* 93 (4): 475–86.

Ling, W., R. A. Rawson, and M. A. Compton. 1994. Substitution pharmacotherapies for opioid addiction: From methadone to LAAM and buprenorphine. *Journal of Psychoactive Drugs* 26 (2): 119–28.

Ling, W., D. R. Wesson, and D. E. Smith. 2005. Prescription opiate abuse. In *Substance abuse: A comprehensive textbook,* 4th ed., eds. J. H. Lowinson, P. Ruiz, R. B. Millman, and J. G. Langrod, 459–68. Philadelphia, PA: Lippincott Williams and Wilkins.

London, E. D., M. Ernst, S. Grant, K. Bonson, and A. Weinstein. 2000. Orbitofrontal cortex and human drug abuse: Functional imaging. *Cerebral Cortex* 10:334–42.

Longo, L. P., T. Parran, B. Johnson, and W. Kinsey. 2000. Addiction: Part II. Identification and management of the drug-seeking patient. *American Family Physician* 61:2401–8.

Loperamide package insert. 2006. Teva Pharmaceuticals USA. Revised 10/2006. Available at: http://dailymed.nlm.nih.gov/dailymed/drugInfo.cfm?id=2387.

Luty, J. 2003. What works in drug addiction? *Advances in Psychiatric Treatment* 9:280–88.

Maddux, J. F. 1978. History of the hospital treatment programs, 1935–1974. In *Drug addiction and the U.S. Public Health Service,* eds. W. R. Martin and H. Isbell. DHEW Publ. No. (ADM) 77-434. Washington, DC: U.S. Government Printing Office.

Maddux, J. F., and D. P. Desmond. 1981. *Careers of opioid users.* New York: Praeger.

Magura, S., S. J. Lee, E. A. Salsitz, A. Kolodny, S. D. Whitley, T. Taubes, R. Seewald, H. Joseph, D. J. Kayman, C. Fong, L. A. Marsch, and A. Rosenblum. 2007. Outcomes of buprenorphine maintenance in office-based practice. *Journal of Addictive Diseases* 26 (2): 13–23.

Magura, S., and A. Rosenblum. 2000. Leaving methadone treatment: Lessons learned, lessons forgotten, lessons ignored. *Mount Sinai Journal of Medicine* 67 (5 and 6): 62–64.

———. 2001. Leaving methadone treatment: Lessons learned, lessons forgotten, lessons ignored. *Mount Sinai Journal of Medicine* 68 (1): 62–74.

Mahowald, M. L., J. A. Singh, and P. Majeski. 2005. Opioid use by patients in an orthopedics spine clinic. *Arthritis and Rheumatism* 52:312–21.

Manchikanti, L. 2006. Prescription drug abuse: What is being done to address this new drug epidemic? Testimony before the Subcommittee on Criminal Justice, Drug Policy and Human Resources. *Pain Physician* 9:287–321.

———. 2007. National drug control policy and prescription drug abuse: Facts and fallacies. *Pain Physician* 10:399–424.

Manchikanti, L., K. R. Brown, and V. Singh. 2002. National All Schedules Prescription Electronic Reporting Act (NASPER): Balancing substance abuse and medical necessity. *Pain Physician* 5:294–319.

Manchikanti, L., and A. Singh. 2008. Therapeutic opioids: A ten-year perspective on the complexities and complications of the escalating use, abuse, and nonmedical use of opioids. Opioid special issue, *Pain Physician* 11: S63–88.

Mansbach, R. S., and R. A. Moore Jr. 2006. Formulation considerations for the development of medications with abuse potential. *Drug and Alcohol Dependence* 83 (Suppl 1): S15–22.

Martell, B. A., P. G. O'Connor, R. D. Kerns, W. C. Becker, K. H. Morales, T. R. Kosten, and D. A. Fiellin. 2007. Systematic review: Opioid treatment for chronic back pain: Prevalence, efficacy, and association with addiction. *Annals of Internal Medicine* 146 (2): 116–27.

Martin, W. R., and D. R. Jasinski. 1969. Physiological parameters of morphine dependence in man: Tolerance, early abstinence, protracted abstinence. *Journal of Psychiatric Research* 7:9–17.

Mattick, R. P., C. Breen, J. Kimber, and M. Davoli. 2003. Methadone maintenance therapy versus no opioid replacement therapy for opioid dependence. *Cochrane Database of Systematic Reviews* (2): CD002209.

Mattison, J. B. 1885. *The treatment of opium addiction.* New York: G. P. Putnam's Sons.

McAleer, S. D., R. J. Mills, T. Polack, T. Hussain, P. E. Rolan, A. D. Gibbs, F. G. Mullins, and Z. Hussein. 2003. Pharmacokinetics of high-dose buprenorphine following single administration of sublingual tablet formulations in opioid naïve healthy male volunteers under a naltrexone block. *Drug and Alcohol Dependence* 72 (1): 75–83.

McCabe, S. E., and C. J. Boyd. 2005. Sources of prescription drugs for illicit use. *Addictive Behaviors* 30 (7): 1342–50.

McCabe, S. E., C. J. Boyd, J. A. Cranford, and C. J. Teter. 2009. Motives for nonmedical use of prescription opioids among high school seniors in the United States: Self-treatment and beyond. *Archives of Pediatrics and Adolescent Medicine* 163 (8): 739–44.

McCabe, S. E., C. J. Boyd, and C. J. Teter. 2006. Medical use, illicit use, and diversion of abusable prescription drugs. *Journal of American College Health* 54 (5): 269–78.

McCabe, S. E., C. J. Boyd, and A. Young. 2007. Medical and nonmedical use of prescription drugs among secondary school students. *Journal of Adolescent Health* 40 (1): 76–83.

McCabe, S. E., C. J. Teter, C. J. Boyd, J. R. Knight, and H. Wechsler. 2005. Nonmedical use of prescription opioids among U.S. college students: Prevalence and correlates from a national survey. *Addictive Behaviors* 30 (4): 789–805.

McCance-Katz, E. F., M. N. Gourevitch, J. Arnsten, J. Sarlo, P. Rainey, and P. Jatlow. 2002. Modified directly observed therapy (MDOT) for injection drug users with HIV disease. *American Journal on Addictions* 11 (4): 271–78.

McCance-Katz, E. F., P. M. Rainey, P. Smith, G. Morse, G. Friedland, M. Gourevitch, and P. Jatlow. 2004. Drug interactions between opioid and antiretroviral medications: Interaction between methadone, LAAM, and nelfinavir. *American Journal on Addictions* 13:163–80.

McCaskill, C. 2002. Oversight controls in the state's Medicaid prescription drug program, April 18. *Performance Audit Report* No. 2002–29, 4. Cited in Prescription drug abuse: What is being done to address this new drug epidemic? Testimony before the Subcommittee on Criminal Justice, Drug Policy and Human Resources by L. Manchikanti. *Pain Physician* 9 (2006): 287–321.

McGlothlin, W. H., M. D. Anglin, and B. D. Wilson. 1977. An evaluation of the California Civil Addict Program. NIDA Services Research Monograph Series. DHEW Publication No. (ADM) 78-558. Washington, DC: U.S. Government Printing Office.

McLellan, A. T. 1983. Patient characteristics associated with outcome. In *Research on the treatment of narcotic addiction: State of the art,* eds. J. R. Cooper, F. Altman, B. S. Brown, and D. Czechowicz. Rockville, MD: National Institute on Drug Abuse.

McLellan, A. T., G. S. Skipper, M. Campbell, and R. L. DuPont. 2008. Five-year outcomes in a cohort study of physicians treated for substance use disorders in the United States. *British Medical Journal* 337:a2038.

Meier, B. 2001. Overdoses of painkiller are linked to 282 deaths. *New York Times,* December 10.

———. 2003. The delicate balance of pain and addiction. *New York Times,* November 25.

Meier, B., and M. Peterson. 2001. Sales of painkiller grew rapidly, but success brought a high cost. *New York Times,* March 5.

Methadone Anonymous. 2007a. History of MA. Available at: www.methadone-anonymous.org.

Methadone Anonymous. 2007b. MA home page. Available at: www.methadone-anonymous.org.

Miller, N. S., and A. Greenfeld. 2004. Patient characteristics and risks factors for development of dependence on hydrocodone and oxycodone. *American Journal of Therapeutics* 11:26–32.

Minozzi, S., L. Amato, S. Vecchi, U. Kirchmayer, and A. Verster. 2006. Oral naltrexone maintenance treatment for opioid dependence. *Cochrane Database of Systematic Reviews* (1): CD001333.

Mintzer, S. 2002. Cognitive impairment in methadone maintenance patients. *Drug and Alcohol Dependence* 67 (1): 41–51.

Moolchan, E. T., A. Umbricht, and D. Epstein. 2001. Therapeutic drug monitoring in methadone maintenance: Choosing a matrix. *Journal of Addictive Diseases* 20:55–73.

Moore, B. A., D. A. Fiellin, D. T. Barry, L. E. Sullivan, M. C. Chawarski, P. G. O'Connor, and R. S. Schottenfeld. 2007. Primary care office-based buprenorphine treatment: Comparison of heroin and prescription opioid dependent patients. *Journal of General Internal Medicine* 22:527–30.

Morgan, H. W. 1974. *Drugs in America: A social history 1800–1980.* New York: Syracuse University Press.

Muir, H. 2006. Abuse of prescription drugs fuelled by online recipes. *New Scientist* 2554, June 5.

Musto, D. F. 1974. Early history of heroin in the United States. In *Addiction,* ed. P. G. Bourne. New York: Academic Press.

———. 1987. *The American disease: Origins of narcotic control.* New York: Oxford University Press.

———. 1991. Opium, cocaine and marijuana in American history. *Scientific American* (July): 20–27.

———. 1999. *The American disease: Origins of narcotic control.* 3rd. ed. New York: Oxford University Press.

Narcotics Anonymous. 1992. *An introductory guide to Narcotics Anonymous.* Revised. Narcotics Anonymous World Services. www.na.org.

———. 2010. Facts about NA. NA World Services. www.na.org.

National Center on Addiction and Substance Abuse at Columbia University (CASA). 2005. *Under the counter: The diversion and abuse of controlled prescription drugs in the U.S.* New York: CASA. Available at: www.casacolumbia.org. Cited in Prescription drug abuse: What is being done to address this new drug epidemic? Testimony before the Subcommittee on Criminal Justice, Drug Policy and Human Resources by L. Manchikanti. *Pain Physician* 9 (2006): 287–321.

———. 2007. "You've got drugs" IV: Prescription drug pushers on the Internet. New York: CASA. Available at: www.casacolumbia.org. Cited in Prescription opioid abuse and diversion in an urban community: The results of an ultrarapid assessment by J. A. Inciardi, H. L. Surratt, T. J. Cicero, and R. A. Beard. *Pain Medicine* 10 (3): 537–48.

———. 2008. "You've got drugs!" V: Prescription drug pushers on the Internet. New York: CASA. Available at: www.casacolumbia.org.

National Committee Pharmacists Association (NCPA). 1999. NCPA position statements. Medicare reform: JCPP statement, August 10. Available at: www.ncpanet.org/about/ncpa_position_statements/m.shtml#10. Cited in Prescription drug abuse: What is being done to address this new drug epidemic? Testimony before the Subcommittee on Criminal Justice, Drug Policy and Human Resources by L. Manchikanti. *Pain Physician* 9 (2006): 287–321.

National Drug Intelligence Center (NDIC). 2007. *Methadone diversion, abuse, and misuse: Deaths increasing at alarming rate.* Product No. 2007-Q0317-001. Available at: www.justice.gov/ndic/pubs25/25930/index.htm.

———. 2009. *National prescription drug threat assessment 2009.* Document ID: 2009-L0487-001. Available at: www.justice.gov/ndic/pubs33/33775/index.htm.

National Institute on Drug Abuse. 2010. *Heroin.* NIDA InfoFacts. Available at: www.nida.nih.gov/infofacts/heroin.html.

National Institutes of Health (NIH). 1997. *Effective medical treatment of opiate addiction. NIH consensus statement* 15 (6): 1–38.

Nebraska State Historical Society. 2005. Keeley cure. Available at: www.nebraskahistory.org/publish/publicat/timeline/keeley_cure.htm.

New York Times. 2009. Ban on painkiller Darvon is recommended to F.D.A. Associated Press. January 31.

Noda, Y., and T. Nabeshima. 2004. Opiate physical dependence and N-methyl-D-aspartate receptors. *European Journal of Pharmacology* 500:121–28.

Nyswander, M. E. 1956. *The drug addict as a patient.* New York: Grune and Stratton.

O'Donnell, J. A. 1969. *Narcotics addicts in Kentucky.* U.S. Public Health Service Publication No. 1881. Chevy Chase, MD: National Institute of Mental Health. Cited in *Licit and illicit drugs: The consumers union report on narcotics, stimulants, depressants, inhalants, hallucinogens, and marijuana—including caffeine, nicotine, and alcohol* by E. M. Brecher and the editors of *Consumer Reports.* Boston: Little, Brown and Company, 1972.

Office of National Drug Control Policy (ONDCP). 2004. *The economic costs of drug abuse in the United States, 1992–2002.* Washington, DC: Executive Office of the President. Available at: http://staging.whitehousedrugpolicy.gov/Publications/economic_costs.

Oldendorf, W. H. 1992. Some relationships between addiction and drug delivery to the brain. In *Bioavailabilty of drugs to the brain and the blood-brain barrier,* volume 120, eds. J. Frankenheim and R. M. Brown. Rockville, MD: National Institute on Drug Abuse. Cited in Can abuse deterrent formulations make a difference? Expectation and speculation by S. H. Budman, J. M. G. Serrano, and S. F. Butler. *Harm Reduction Journal* 6 (2009): 8–15.

Otton, S. V., M. Schadel, S. W. Cheung, H. L. Kaplan, U. E. Busto, and E. M. Sellers. 1993. CYP 2D6 phenotype determines the metabolic conversion of hydrocodone to hydromorphone. *Clinical Pharmacology and Therapeutics* 54:463–72.

Ouimette, P. C., R. Moos, and J. Finney. 1998. Influence of outpatient treatment and 12-step group involvement on one year substance abuse outcomes. *Journal of Studies on Alcohol* 59:513–22.

Package insert. 2006. G.D. Searle. Revised 4/2006. Available at: www.pfizer.com/pfizer/download/uspi_lomotil.pdf.

Parran, T. 1997. Prescription drug abuse. A question of balance. *Medical Clinics of North America* 8:967–78.

Pasierb, S. J. 2006. Testimony of Stephen J. Pasierb, president and CEO, Partnership for a Drug-Free America, before the house Subcommittee on Criminal Justice, Drug Policy and Human Resources, July 26. Cited in Prescription drug abuse: What is being done to address this new drug epidemic? Testimony before the Subcommittee on Criminal Justice, Drug Policy and Human Resources by L. Manchikanti. *Pain Physician* 9 (2006): 287–321.

Passik, S. D. 2009. Issues in long-term opioid therapy: Unmet needs, risks, and solutions. *Mayo Clinic Proceedings* 84 (7): 593–601.

Paulozzi, L. J., D. S. Budnitz, and Y. Xi. 2006. Increasing deaths from opioid analgesics in the United States. *Pharmacoepidemiology and Drug Safety* 15 (9): 618–27.

Pergolizzi, J. V., R. B. Raffa, and E. Gould. 2009. Considerations on the use of oxymorphone in geriatric patients. *Expert Opinion on Drug Safety* 8 (5): 603–13.

Pepper, W. 1886. *System of practical medicine.* Cited in *Licit and illicit drugs: The consumers union report on narcotics, stimulants, depressants, inhalants, hallucinogens, and marijuana—including caffeine, nicotine, and alcohol* by E. M. Brecher and the editors of *Consumer Reports.* Boston: Little, Brown and Company, 1972.

Pharo, G. H., and L. Zhou. 2005. Pharmacologic management of cancer pain. *Journal of the American Osteopathic Association* 11 (Suppl 5): S21–29.

PhRMA. 2002. Code on the interactions with healthcare professionals. Pharmaceutical Research and Manufacturers of America, July. Available at: www.phrma.org/code_on_interactions_with_healthcare_professionals.

Pills Anonymous. 2010. www.pillsanonymous.org.

Potter, J. S., G. Hennessy, J. A. Borrow, S. F. Greenfield, and R. D. Weiss. 2004. Substance use histories in patients seeking treatment for controlled-release oxycodone dependence. *Drug and Alcohol Dependence* 76 (2): 213–15.

Poyhia, R., T. Seppala, K. T. Olkkola, and E. Kalso. 1992. The pharmacokinetics and metabolism of oxycodone after intramuscular and oral administration to healthy subjects. *British Journal of Clinical Pharmacology* 33:617–21.

Prommer, E. 2006. Oxymorphone: A review. *Supportive Care in Cancer* 14:109–15.

———. 2007. Levorphanol: The forgotten opioid. *Supportive Care in Cancer* 15 (3): 259–64.

Rannazzisi, J. T. 2006. Testimony of Joseph T. Rannazzisi, deputy assistant administrator, Office of Diversion Control, Drug Enforcement Administration, U.S. Department of Justice, before the Subcommittee on Criminal Justice, Drug Policy and Human Resources, July 26. Cited in Prescription drug abuse: What is being done to address this new drug epidemic? Testimony before the Subcommittee on Criminal Justice, Drug Policy and Human Resources by L. Manchikanti. *Pain Physician* 9 (2006): 287–321.

Rapeli, P., D. Fabitius, H. Alho, M. Salaspuro, K. Wahlbeck, and H. Kalska. 2007. Methadone vs. buprenorphine/naloxone during early opioid substitution treatment: A naturalistic comparison of cognitive performance relative to healthy controls. *BMC Clinical Pharmacology* 7:5.

Rehman, Z. 2001. Opioid abuse. *eMedicine* August 15, 2 (8) section 2. Cited in National All Schedules Prescription Electronic Reporting Act (NASPER): Balancing substance abuse and medical necessity by L. Manchikanti, K. R. Brown, and V. Singh. *Pain Physician* 5:294–319.

Reisinger, M. 2006. Injecting buprenorphine tablets: A manageable risk. *Heroin Addiction and Related Clinical Problems* 8 (4): 29–40.

Rettig, R. A., and A. Yarmolinsky, eds. 1995. *Federal regulation of methadone treatment.* Institute of Medicine. Washington, DC: National Academy Press.

Robinson, T. E., and K. C. Berridge. 2000. The psychology and neurobiology of addiction: An incentive-sensitization view. *Addiction* 95 (Suppl 2): S91–117.

Rogers, R. D., and T. W. Robbins. 2001. Investigating the neurocognitive deficits associated with chronic drug misuse. *Current Opinion in Neurobiology* 11:250–57.

Rolls, E. T. 1996. The orbitofrontal cortex. *Philosophical Transactions of the Royal Society of London, Series B, Biological Sciences* 351:1433–43.

Rosenberg, D. 2001. Now the abuse is an epidemic. *Newsweek,* April 9.

Rosenblum, A., M. Parrino, S. H. Schnoll, C. Fong, C. Maxwell, C. M. Cleland, S. Magura, and J. D. Haddox. 2007. Prescription opioid abuse among enrollees into methadone maintenance treatment. *Drug and Alcohol Dependence* 90:64–71.

Sarhill, N., D. Walsh, and K. A. Nelson. 2001. Hydromorphone: Pharmacology and clinical applications in cancer patients. *Supportive Care in Cancer* 9:84–96.

Schifano, F., G. Zamparutti, F. Zambello, A. Oyefeso, P. Deluca, M. Balestrieri, D. Little, and A. H. Ghodse. 2006. Review of deaths related to analgesic- and cough suppressant-opioids; England and Wales 1996–2002. *Pharmacopsychiatry* 39 (5): 185–91.

Schmitz, R. 1985. Friedrich Wilhelm Sertürner and the discovery of morphine. *Pharmacy in History* 27:61–74.

Schwartz, R. H. 1998. Adolescent heroin use: A review. *Pediatrics* 102:1461–66.

Sees, K. L., M. E. Di Marino, N. K. Ruediger, C. T. Sweeney, and S. Shiffman. 2005. Non-medical use of OxyContin tablets in the United States. *Journal of Pain and Palliative Care Pharmacotherapy* 19 (2): 13–23.

Senay, E. 1984. Clinical implications of drug abuse treatment outcome research. In *Drug abuse treatment evaluation,* eds. F. M. Tims, F. Ludford, and J. P. Ludford. Rockville, MD: National Institute on Drug Abuse.

Shaffer, L. 1995. *Synanon's history and influence in therapeutic communities and emotional growth schools.* Sandpoint, ID: Woodbury Reports. Available at: www.strugglingteens .com/archives/1995/2/oe05.html.

Shaham, Y., S. Erb, and J. Stewart. 2000. Stress-induced relapse to heroin and cocaine seeking in rats: A review. *Brain Research Reviews* 33 (1): 13–33.

Sheeren, M. 1988. The relationship between relapse and involvement in Alcoholics Anonymous. *Journal of Studies on Alcohol* 49:104–6.

Shirer, M. Forrester Technographics finds that young consumers are internalizing net rules. Available at: www.forrester.com/ER/Press/Release/0,1769,158,FF.html (Accessed March 8, 2000). Cited in Internet and psychoactive substance use among innovative drug users by E. W. Boyer, M. Shannon, and P. L. Hibberd. *Pediatrics* 115 (2005):302–5.

Silverman, S. M. 2009. Opioid induced hyperalgesia: Clinical implications for the pain practitioner. *Pain Physician* 12:679–84.

Simoni-Wastila, L., and G. Strickler. 2004. Risk factors associated with problem use of prescription drugs. *American Journal of Public Health* 94:266–69.

Simpson, D. D., and S. B. Sells. 1982. Effectiveness of treatment for drug abuse: An overview of the DARP research program. *Advances in Alcohol and Substance Abuse* 2:7–29.

Smith, H. S. 2008. Opioid-related issues "popping" up again. *Pain Physician* 11:S1–4.

Smithsonian National Museum of American History. n.d. Origin of patent medicines. Available at: http://americanhistory.si.edu/collections/group_detail.cfm?key=1253gkey =51&page=2.

Specka, M., T. Finkbeiner, E. Lodemann, K. Leifert, J. Kluwig, and M. Gastpar. 2000. Cognitive-motor performance of methadone-maintained patients. *European Addiction Research* 6:8–19.

Spiller, H., D. J. Lorenz, E. J. Bailey, and R. C. Dart. 2009. Epidemiological trends in abuse and misuse of prescription opioids. *Journal of Addictive Diseases* 28 (2): 130–36.

Sproule, B., B. Brands, S. Li, and L. Catz-Biro. 2009. Changing patterns in opioid addiction: Characterizing users of oxycodone and other opioids. *Canadian Family Physician* 55 (1): 68–69.

Stephens, R. C. 1991. *The street addict role: A theory of heroin addiction.* Albany: State University of New York Press.

Stinchfield, R., and P. Owen. 1998. Hazelden's model of treatment and its outcome. *Addictive Behaviors* 23 (5): 669–83.

Strassels, S. A. 2009. Economic burden of prescription opioid misuse and abuse. *Journal of Managed Care Pharmacy* 15 (7): 556–62.

Streltzer, J., P. Ziegler, and B. Johnson. 2009. American Academy of Addiction Psychiatry. Cautionary guidelines for the use of opioids in chronic pain. *American Journal on Addictions* 18 (1): 1–4.

Subramaniam, G. A., and M. A. Stitzer. 2009. Clinical characteristics of treatment-seeking prescription opioid vs. heroin-using adolescents with opioid use disorder. *Drug and Alcohol Dependence* 101 (1-2): 13–19.

Substance Abuse and Mental Health Services Administration (SAMHSA), Office of Applied Studies. 2004. *The DAWN report: Benzodiazepines in drug abuse-related emergency department visits: 1995–2002.* April.

———. 2005. *Results from the 2004 National Survey on Drug Use and Health: National findings.* NSDUH Series H-28, DHHS Publication No. SMA 05-4062.

———. 2006a. *The DASIS report: Non-heroin opiate admissions: 2003.* Issue 14.

———. 2006b. *The DAWN report: Opiate-related drug misuse deaths in six states: 2003.* Issue 19.

———. 2006c. *The NSDUH report: How young adults obtain prescription pain relievers for nonmedical use.* Issue 39.

———. 2007a. *Results from the 2006 National Survey on Drug Use and Health: National findings.* NSDUH Series H-32, DHHS Publication No. SMA 07-4293. Cited in Prescription opioid abuse and diversion in an urban community: The results of an ultrarapid assessment by J. A. Inciardi, H. L. Surratt, T. J. Cicero, and R. A. Beard. *Pain Medicine* 2009 10 (3): 537–48.

———. 2007b. *National Survey of Substance Abuse Treatment Services (N-SSATS): 2006. Data on Substance Abuse Treatment Facilities,* DASIS Series: S-39, DHHS Publication No. (SMA) 07-4296.

———. 2007c. *The NSDUH report: Patterns and trends in nonmedical prescription pain reliever use: 2002 to 2005.* April 6.

———. 2010. *The TEDS report: Substance abuse treatment admissions involving abuse of pain relievers: 1998 and 2008.* July 15.

Suleman, R., H. Abourjaily, and M. Rosenberg. 2002. OxyContin: Misuse and abuse. *Journal of the Massachusetts Dental Society* 51:56–58.

Suler, J. 1998. *Psychology of cyberspace: Adolescents in cyberspace.* Lawrenceville, NJ: Rider University. Cited in Internet and psychoactive substance use among innovative drug users by E. W. Boyer, M. Shannon, and P. L. Hibberd. *Pediatrics* 115 (2005): 302–5.

Sullum, J. 2004. Pill stoppers: The DEA acknowledges yet denies the conflict between drug control and pain control. *Reason Magazine,* August 20. Available at: http://reason.com/archives/2004/08/20/pill-stoppers.

Sung, H. E., L. Richter, R. Vaughan, P. B. Johnson, and B. Thom. 2005. Nonmedical use of prescription opioids among teenagers in the United States: Trends and correlates. *Journal of Adolescent Health* 37 (1): 44–51.

Sunshine, A., R. Axtmayer, N. Z. Olson, E. Laska, and I. Ramos. 1988. Analgesic efficacy of pentazocine versus a pentazocine-naloxone combination following oral administration. *Clinical Journal of Pain* 4:35–40.

Szalavitz, M. 2001. Web sites and misinformation about illicit drugs. *New England Journal of Medicine* 345:1710.

———. 2004. Dr. Feelscared: Drug warriors put the fear of prosecution in physicians who dare to treat pain. *Reason Magazine,* August. Available at: http://reason.com/archives/2004/08/01/dr-feelscared.

Terry, C. E., and M. Pellens. 1928. *The opium problem.* New York: Committee on Drug Addictions, Bureau of Social Hygiene. Cited in *Licit and illicit drugs: The consumers union report on narcotics, stimulants, depressants, inhalants, hallucinogens, and marijuana—including caffeine, nicotine, and alcohol* by E. M. Brecher and the editors of *Consumer Reports.* Boston: Little, Brown and Company, 1972.

Tharp, A. M., R. E. Winecker, and D. C. Winston. 2004. Fatal intravenous fentanyl abuse: Four cases involving extraction of fentanyl from transdermal patches. *American Journal of Forensic Medicine and Pathology* 25:178–81.

Thorpe, S. J., E. T. Rolls, and S. Maddison. 1983. The orbitofrontal cortex: Neuronal activity in the behaving monkey. *Experimental Brain Research* 49:93–115.

Threlkeld, M., T. Parran, C. Adelman, S. Grey, and J. Yu. 2006. Tramadol versus buprenorphine for the management of acute heroin withdrawal: A retrospective cohort controlled study. *American Journal on Addiction* 15:186–91.

Time Magazine, 1939. Medicine: Keeley Cure. September 25.

Tims, F. M., N. Jainchill, and G. De Leon. 1994. Therapeutic communities and treatment research. *Therapeutic community: Advances in research and application,* NIDA Research Monograph 144.

Tough, P. 2001. The alchemy of OxyContin. *New York Times,* July 29.

Toumbourou, J. W., and M. Hamilton. 2003. *The early impact of involvement in Narcotics Anonymous self-help groups. A report from the Role of Self-Help Groups in Drug Treatment Research Project.* Fitzroy, Australia: Turning Point Alcohol and Drug Centre.

Towns, C. B. 1912. Peril of the drug habit. *Century Magazine* 84:580–87. Cited in *Licit and illicit drugs: The consumers union report on narcotics, stimulants, depressants, inhalants, hallucinogens, and marijuana—including caffeine, nicotine, and alcohol* by E. M. Brecher and the editors of *Consumer Reports.* Boston: Little, Brown and Company, 1972.

Trescot, A. M., M. V. Boswell, S. L. Atluri, H. C. Hansen, T. R. Deer, S. Abdi, J. F. Jasper, V. Singh, A. E. Jordan, B. W. Johnson, R. S. Cicala, E. E. Dunbar, S. Helm 2nd, K. G. Varley, P. K. Suchdev, J. R. Swicegood, A. K. Calodney, B. A. Ogoke, W. S. Minore, and L. Manchikanti. 2006. Opioid guidelines in the management of chronic non-cancer pain. *Pain Physician* 9:1–39.

Trescot, A. M., S. Datta, M. Lee, and H. Hansen. 2008. Opioid pharmacology. *Pain Physician* 11:S133–53.

Tso, P. H., and Y. H. Wong. 2003. Molecular basis of opioid dependence: Role of signal regulation by G-proteins. *Clinical and Experimental Pharmacology and Physiology* 30:307–16.

Ulyankina, T. I. 1987. A history of opium remedies and the emerging problem of drug addiction. In *Alcoholism and Non-Alcohol Toxicomanias. Collection of research papers,* ed. I. N. Pyatnitskaya. Moscow Publishing House of the 2nd Moscow State Medicial Institute, 175–86. Cited in *Licit and illicit drugs: The consumers union report on narcotics, stimulants, depressants, inhalants, hallucinogens, and marijuana—including caffeine, nicotine, and alcohol* by E. M. Brecher and the editors of *Consumer Reports.* Boston: Little, Brown and Company, 1972.

U.S. Department of Health and Human Services (US DHHS). 2001. OxyContin: Prescription drug abuse. *CSAT Advisory* 1(1).

U.S. General Accounting Office (USGAO). 2000. Internet pharmacies: Adding disclosure would aid state and federal oversight. GAO Publication No. GAO-01-69, October.

————. 2003. OxyContin abuse and diversion and efforts to address the problem. Washington, DC: U.S. Government Printing Office; Dec. 2003 Report to Congressional Requesters, GAO Publication No. GAO-04-110. Cited in Prescription opioid abuse and diversion in an urban community: The results of an ultrarapid assessment by J. A. Inciardi, H. L. Surratt, T. J. Cicero, and R. A. Beard. *Pain Medicine* 10 (3): 537–48.

————. 2009. Methadone-associated overdose deaths: Factors contributing to increased deaths and efforts to prevent them. March. Available at: www.gao.gov/new.items/ d09341.pdf.

van den Brink, W., and C. Haasen. 2006. Evidenced-based treatment of opioid-dependent patients. *Canadian Journal of Psychiatry* 51:635–46.

van den Brink, W., and J. M. van Ree. 2003. Pharmacological treatments for heroin and cocaine addiction. *European Neuropsychopharmacology* 13:476–87.

van Ness, P. H., W. R. Davis, and B. D. Johnson. 2004. Socioeconomic marginality and health services utilization among Central Harlem substance users. *Substance Use and Misuse* 39 (1): 61–85.

Vederhus, J. K., and Ø. Kristensen. 2006. High effectiveness of self-help programs after drug addiction therapy. *BMC Psychiatry* 6:35.

Verdejo, A., I. Toribio, C. Orozco, K. L. Puente, and M. Pérez-García. 2005. Neuropsychological functioning in methadone maintenance patients versus abstinent heroin abusers. *Drug and Alcohol Dependence* 78 (3): 283–88.

Vogel, H. S., E. Knight, A. B. Laudet, and S. Magura. 1998. Double Trouble in Recovery: Self-help for the dually diagnosed. *Psychiatric Rehabilitation Journal* 21:356–64.

Volinn, E., J. D. Fargo, and P. G. Fine. 2009. Opioid therapy for nonspecific low back pain and the outcome of chronic work loss. *Pain* 142 (3): 194–201.

Volkow, N. D. 2006. Testimony of Nora D. Volkow, M.D., director, National Institute on Drug Abuse, National Institutes of Health, U.S. Department of Health and Human Services. Before the Subcommittee on Criminal Justice, Drug Policy, and Human Resources Committee, July 26. Cited in Prescription drug abuse: What is being done to address this new drug epidemic? Testimony before the Subcommittee on Criminal Justice, Drug Policy and Human Resources by L. Manchikanti. *Pain Physician* 9 (2006): 287–321.

Volkow, N. D., and J. S. Fowler. 2000. Addiction, a disease of compulsion and drive: Involvement of the orbitofrontal cortex. *Cerebral Cortex* 10:318–25.

Vukmir, R. B. 2004. Drug seeking behavior. *American Journal of Drug and Alcohol Abuse* 30:551–75.

Waldorf, D., M. Orlick, and C. Reinarman. 1974. *Morphine Maintenance: The Shreveport Clinic 1919–1923*. Washington, DC: Drug Abuse Council. April. Available at: www.drugpolicy.org/library/morphinecl_library.cfm.

Walsh, S. L., P. A. Nuzzo, M. R. Lofwall, and J. R. Holtman Jr. 2008. The relative abuse liability of oral oxycodone, hydrocodone and hydromorphone assessed in prescription opioid abusers. *Drug and Alcohol Dependence* 98 (3): 191–202.

Walsh, S. L., and K. L. Preston. 1995. Acute administration of buprenorphine in humans: Partial agonist and blockade effects. *Journal of Pharmacology and Experimental Therapeutics* 274:361–72.

Wang, J., and P. J. Christo. 2009. The influence of prescription monitoring programs on chronic pain management. *Pain Physician* 12:507–15.

Warner-Smith, M., S. Darke, M. Lynskey, and W. Hall. 2001. Heroin overdose: Causes and consequences. *Addiction* 96:1113–25.

Washington Physicians Health Program. 2010. Personal communication.

Washton, A. M., M. S. Gold, and A. C. Pottash. 1984. Naltrexone in addicted physicians and business executives. *NIDA Research Monograph* 55:185–90.

Weathermon, R. A. 1999. Controlled substances diversion: Who attempts it and how. *U.S. Pharmacist* 24 (12): 32–47.

Webster, B. S., M. Cifuentes, S. Verma, and G. Pransky. 2009. Geographic variation in opioid prescribing for acute, work-related, low back pain and associated factors: A multilevel analysis. *American Journal of Industrial Medicine* 52 (2): 162–71.

Webster, L. R., B. Bath, and R. A. Medve. 2009. Opioid formulations in development designed to curtail abuse: Who is the target? *Expert Opinion on Investigational Drugs* 18 (3): 255–63.

Webster, L. R., and R. M. Webster. 2005. Predicting aberrant behaviors in opioid-treated patients: Preliminary validation of the Opioid Risk Tool. *Pain Medicine* 6 (6): 432–42.

Wedam, E. F., G. A. Bigelow, R. E. Johnson, P. A. Nuzzo, and M. C. Haigney. 2007. QT-interval effects of methadone, levomethadyl, and buprenorphine in a randomized trial. *Archives of Internal Medicine* 167 (22): 2469–75.

Weiss, R. D., M. L. Griffin, T. Gallop, L. S. Onken, D. R. Gastfriend, D. Daley, P. Crits-Christoph, S. Bishop, and J. P. Barber. 2000. Self-help group attendance and participation among cocaine dependent patients. *Drug and Alcohol Dependence* 60:169–77.

White, A. G., H. G. Birnbaum, M. N. Mareva, M. Daher, S. Vallow, J. Schein, and N. Katz. 2005. Direct costs of opioid abuse in an insured population in the United States. *Journal of Managed Care Pharmacy* 11 (6): 469–79.

White, A. G., H. G. Birnbaum, M. Shiller, J. Tang, and N. P. Katz. 2009. Analytic models to identify patients at risk for prescription opioid abuse. *American Journal of Managed Care* 15 (12): 897–906.

White, J. M., and R. J. Irvine. 1999. Mechanisms of fatal opioid overdose. *Addiction* 94:961–72.

White, W. L. 1979. Themes in chemical prohibition. In *Drugs in perspective,* 117–82. Rockville, MD: National Institute on Drug Abuse, National Drug Abuse Center.

———. 2009. Addiction medicine in America. In *Principles of addiction medicine,* 4th ed. eds. R. K. Ries, S. Miller, D. A. Fiellin, and R. Saitz. Philadelphia: Lippincott, Williams and Wilkins.

Wilford, B. B. 1990. Abuse of prescription drugs. *Western Journal of Medicine* 152:609–12.

Woolf, C. J., and M. Hashmi. 2004. Use and abuse of opioid analgesics: Potential methods to prevent and deter non-medical consumption of prescription opioids. *Current Opinions in Investigational Drugs* 5:61–66.

World Health Organization (WHO). 1986. WHO's pain relief ladder. Available at: www.who.int/cancer/palliative/painladder/en.

Wunsch, M. J., K. Nakamoto, G. Behonick, and W. Massello. 2009. Opioid deaths in rural Virginia: A description of the high prevalence of accidental fatalities involving prescribed medications. *American Journal on Addictions* 18 (1): 5–14.

Xi, Z. X., and E. A. Stein. 2002. GABAergic mechanisms of opiate reinforcement. *Alcohol and Alcoholism* 37:485–94.

Yablonsky, L. 1969. *Synanon: The tunnel back.* Baltimore, MD: Penguin Books.

———. 1994. *The therapeutic community.* New York: Gardner Press.

Zacny, J. P., S. Gutierrez, and S. A. Bolbolan. 2005. Profiling the subjective, psychomotor, and physiological effects of a hydrocodone/acetaminophen product in recreational drug users. *Drug and Alcohol Dependence* 78:243–52.

Zacny, J. P., and S. A. Lichtor. 2008. Within-subject comparison of the psychopharmacological profiles of oral oxycodone and oral morphine in non-drug-abusing volunteers. *Psychopharmacology* 196 (1): 105–16.

Zafiridis, P. 2001. Mental health and self-help: The paradigm of Narcotics Anonymous (NA) and Alcoholics Anonymous (AA). *Tetradia Psychiatrikis* 73:22–29.

Ziegler, S. J., and N. P. Lovrich Jr. 2003. Pain relief, prescription drugs, and prosecution: A four-state survey of chief prosecutors. *Journal of Law, Medicine, and Ethics* 31:75–100.

INDEX

A

abstinence-based treatment programs.
See Twelve Step programs
abuse
  by adolescents, 3, 64, 66–67, 94–95
  behavioral patterns, 6, 8, 10, 119
  defined, 6
  drug availability and, 70
  potential
    administration route and, 122
    drug classification and, 36–37
    pharmacokinetics and, 121
abuse of prescription opioids
  analgesic potential and, 122–23
  behavioral characteristics, 111
  biological characteristics, 110–11
  costs, 69–70
  factors contributing
    advertising, 95
    criminal activity, 83–86
    diversions, 79–80, 86–90, 87–89
    ease of tampering with formulation, 181
    opioid attractiveness concept, 91, 93–95
    pain management changes, 74–75
    parental unawareness, 95
    patient advocacy groups, 96
    patient behavior, 80–83, 87–90
    sharing with friends/family, 86, 90, 91, 92
    supply networks, 70–74
    treatment by primary care physicians, 76–79, 180
  most frequently, 87
  OxyContin
    attempts to control, 135, 185–86, 188–89
    crime and, 182, 185
    economic factors, 185
    geographic distribution, 182, 184
    personal stories, 182–84
  risk factors, 62–66
  as safe, 65
  signs/symptoms of, 110

abuse-deterrent formulations (ADFs), 133–35
abusers of prescription opioids
  identifiable subgroups, 59–62
  increase in, vii
  non-medical factors affecting, 57–59
  physicians as, 211, 218–19
  prior history of substance abuse, 117, 118, 120
  rate in U.S., 1
  Twelve Step programs specifically for, 199–200
acetaminophen with codeine, street price, 84
acute pain, prescription opioids for, 8
The Addict and the Law (Lindesmith), 50
addiction, 27
  compared to physical dependence, 6–7, 102
  defined, 6, 9
  as disease, 43–45, 97–99, 195–96
  early medical ideas, 27
  as federal crime, 35
  to "feel normal," 105
  iatrogenic, 117–20
  morality and, 30, 31, 97
  nineteenth century understanding of, 30, 31, 43–45
  risk as low for chronic pain treatment, 170–71
  See also opioid addiction
addiction careers, defined, 99
administration routes
  development of abuse-deterrent formulations, 133–36
  factors influencing choice, 123
  of heroin, 26
  of heroin vs. non-heroin opioid users, 68
  high-dose extended-release tablets and abuse, 70
  intravenous injections
    effects of, 110–11, 141
    of hydromorphone, 132–33
    of morphine, 30, 128
    of oxycodone, 131
  methods to alter
    buprenorphine, 123–24
    codeine, 124–25